T0022880

THE ESSENTIAL BOOK OF

CBD

Elements

THE ESSENTIAL BOOK OF

CBD

Transformational healing with cannabidiol

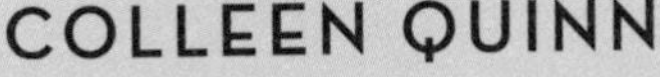

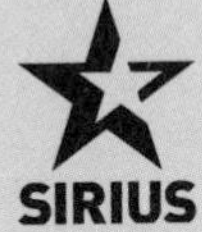

To Donna, Kerrie and Shannon,
for always being my home.

All images courtesy of Shutterstock,
Unsplash and Adobe Stock.

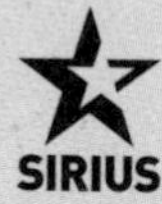

This edition published in 2023 by Sirius Publishing, a division of
Arcturus Publishing Limited,
26/27 Bickels Yard, 151–153 Bermondsey Street,
London SE1 3HA

ISBN: 978-1-3988-2084-5
AD010140UK

Printed in China

Contents

Introduction

I have been blissfully working with, exploring and examining plants and their fascinating chemistry for nearly two decades now. I was contentedly working in the world of aromatherapy and plant science, unaware that there was a plant out there that was going to turn my world upside down. That plant was cannabis. In 2016 cannabis and "her" cannabinoids, especially CBD (only the female plant produces the phytochemicals such as CBD), captured my attention; to this day I continue to be mesmerized by this diversely therapeutic plant.

I had been passionately advocating plant-based skincare, wellness and healthcare solutions for a very long time and, to an extent, I was winning the battle, especially as more and more research became available, and clinical evidence started to support the science and therapeutics of our plants' powerful chemistry. But this path of action got supercharged

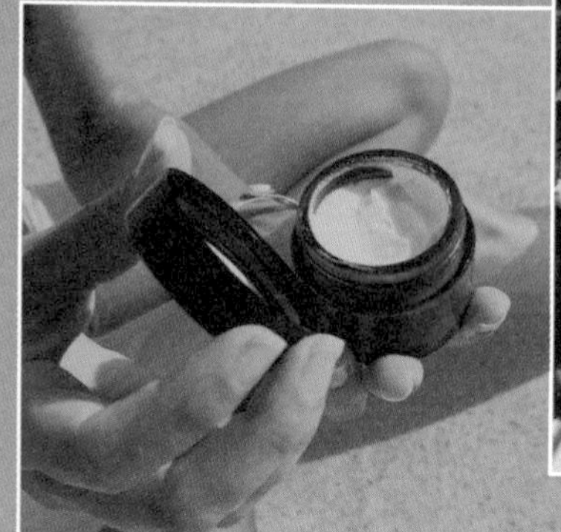

when the world woke up to the healing power of cannabis, its compounds and CBD. A lot of people had heard about CBD long before they heard about cannabis or hemp. Like me, they may have heard about CBD from the remarkable story of Charlotte's web.

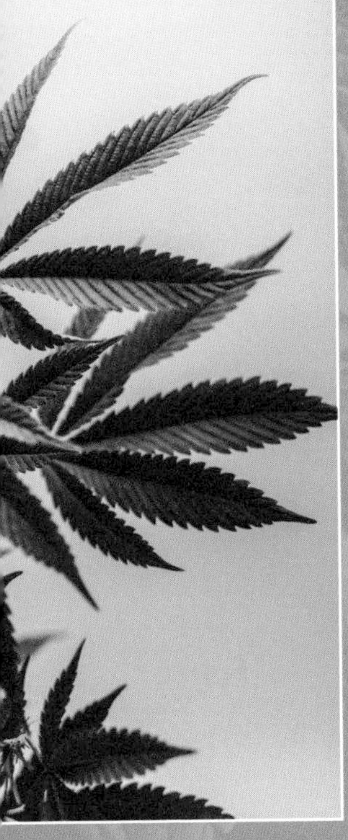

Charlotte's web is a chemovar of cannabis that is strategically cultivated to have very high levels of CBD, as it is created to treat a specific form of childhood epilepsy. The Stanley Brothers, who cultivated the chemovar, began to see successful results with their cannabis plant when it helped a young girl called Charlotte Figi who suffered from Dravet syndrome. Charlotte started to experience a reduction in the frequency of her seizures when she was taking the high-CBD cannabis plant. Charlotte became the inspiration behind the plant's now famous name. To an extent, Charlotte became the face of not just cannabis as a masterful plant medicine, but of the health benefits of this one compound: CBD.

It wasn't until the legalization of cannabis slowly started to open up in North America that I received the opportunity to work with this plant and to understand its chemistry in such a way that I could make formulations and recipes with it at the centre of my scientific yet creative process. For me, the big difference with working with CBD was that it presented an effective solution to an extensive array of conditions and problems. Within the area of wellness and preventive medicine, CBD was proving useful in a way that I had never experienced before with any other plant. I had seen great results when working with various plants synergistically, but cannabis performed brilliantly as a solo solution or when synergized with other plants. I was intrigued!

The longer and deeper I worked with this plant, the more apparent it became to me that, although CBD is not a silver bullet, it is a distinctively therapeutic and effective compound whether we are using it for its anti-inflammatory or antioxidant properties, or utilizing it for our ageing skincare routine, supporting our immune system, helping our muscles to recover, easing into a restful slumber, or supporting us as we manage the daily overwhelming anxiety our busy lives can infect upon us. CBD has quickly become the one plant compound that I, my clients, family and friends, not only need – but are endlessly grateful for.

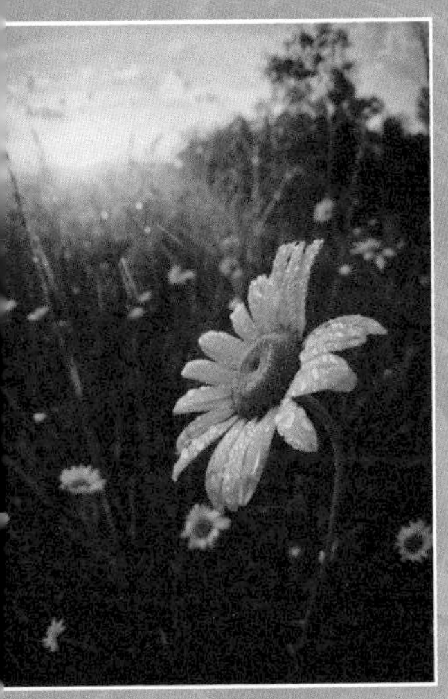

In my experience, the four main areas continually touched upon through a journey of wellness, and which can have the most impact negatively or positively on our daily mood and on how we experience our day are: how we feel pain and stress; the contentment and restfulness we achieve within our sleeping hours; the pleasure, confidence and relaxation we gain from sex; and your health and lifestyle. After years of working with clients and patients, especially terminal patients, so much of our lives are affected by our personal relationship with these four areas of our health and lifestyle: stress, sleep, pain and sex.

I'm a strong believer that if we care for and pay attention to looking after these areas of our health and wellness, we can lead much happier and healthier lives. I've been using CBD as I strive towards thriving within my own journey to consistent wellness and now it's time to share my experiences and learnings with you.

The benefits of CBD are rooted in science, supported by phytochemistry and trusted by millions of beautiful humans who lean on CBD to enhance their daily lives and strengthen their physical and mental health. CBD helps support our immune system, it can decrease anxiety as well as being an influential neuroprotectant, defending and supporting our brain function. It is a formidable anti-inflammatory and antioxidant. CBD is absorbed by our skin and the mucous membrane tissue in our mouth. CBD stimulates a fascinating natural system within our body called the endocannabinoid system. Within the endocannabinoid system, CBD activates a series of actions beneficial to our health.

In this book you will learn about CBD – the plant itself, the compound, the chemistry, its impressive therapeutic properties, and the system within your body that it feeds. You will go from feeling confused about CBD and how to use it, to feeling confident in your understanding and knowledge around how it works within your body and how you can use it for the betterment of your health. You will explore the four areas of wellness that I have found to be fundamental to growing towards being a healthy formidable human. We look at why these specific areas are so important and what we need to know about them physiologically to feel empowered and enlightened about our own health.

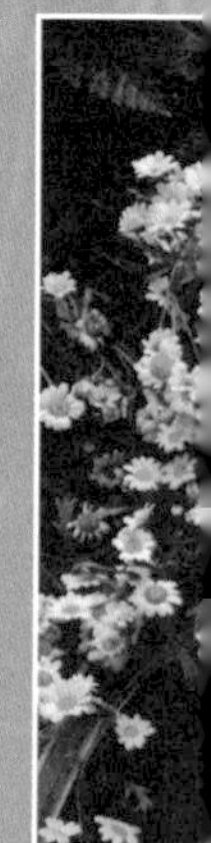

Without action the knowledge and education you will gain within these pages are only words, so I have created 12 recipes for you that are rich in CBD, essential oils and other botanicals. These you can make in your own kitchen and use every day to support your health. Whether you need support sleeping, relief for aching joints or some aphrodisiac encouragement, I have considered all. In the recipe chapter I walk you through each recipe to enable you to use CBD to take control of your personal wellness journey.

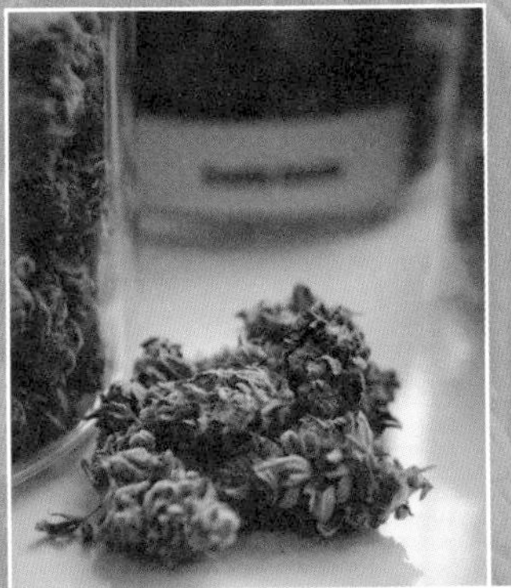

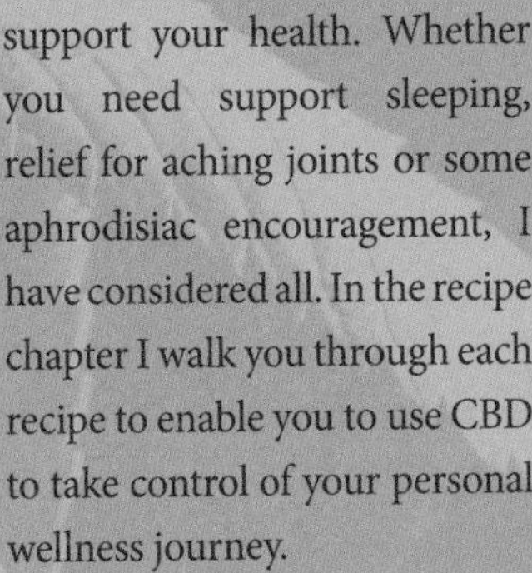

The main question I get asked about CBD is, "how can CBD make me healthier and happier?" My intention with this book is to answer that question.

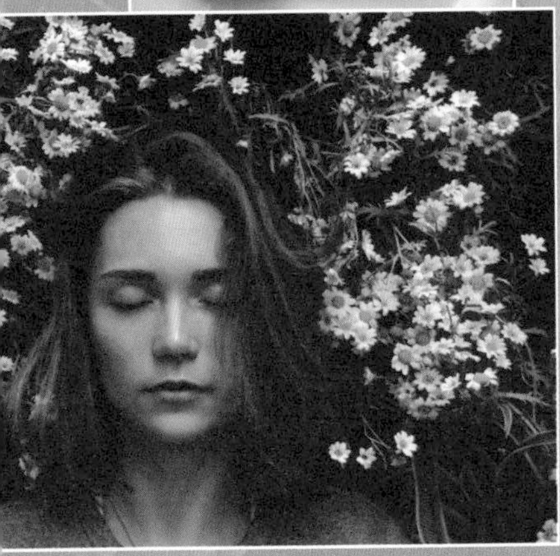

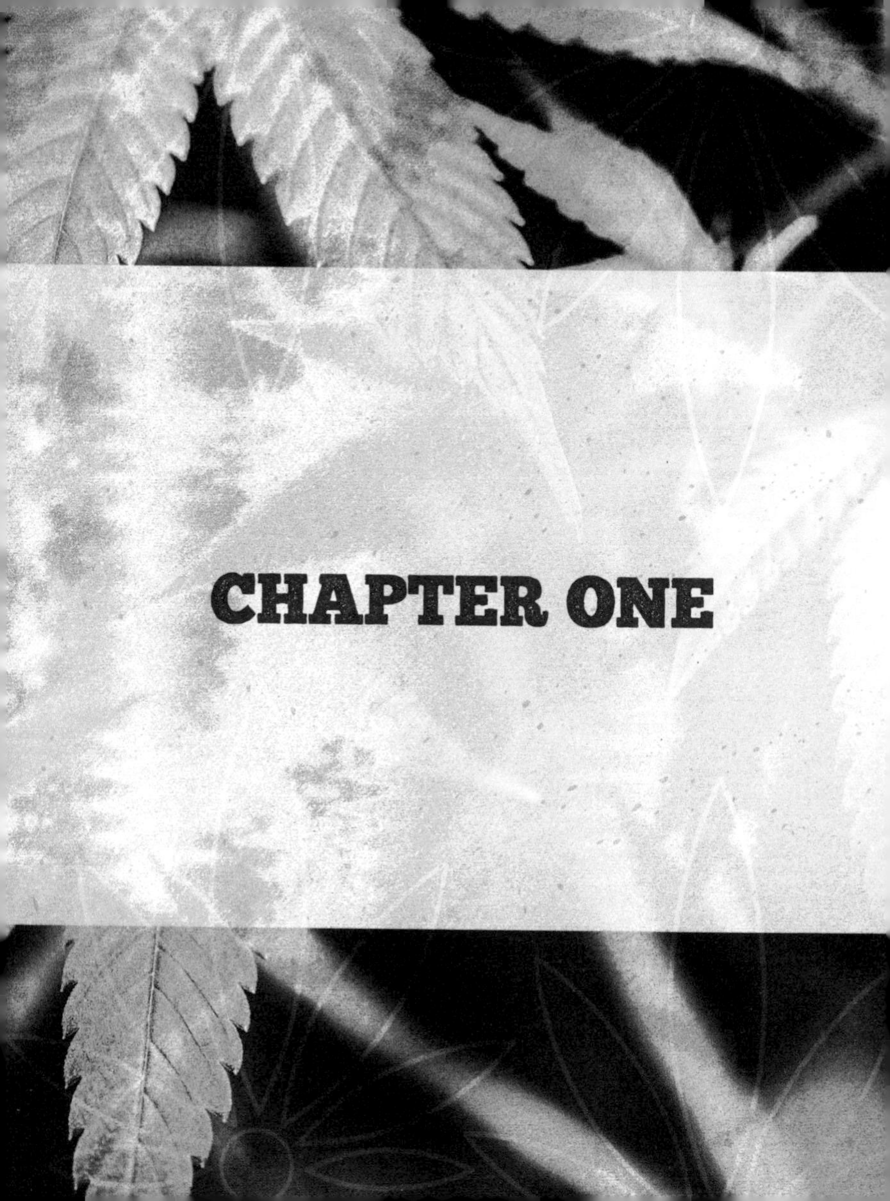

CHAPTER ONE

What is CBD?

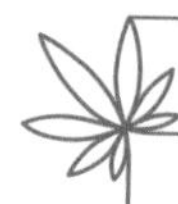

It is impossible to build anything solid without foundations. In this case our foundations are gaining an understanding of what CBD is, how it works inside the body, and how we can use it for the betterment of our health, physically, mentally and emotionally.

Cannabidiol (CBD) is considered to be one of the most effective parts of the hemp plant, used for a wide variety of therapeutic properties. Various types of inflammation, including digestive disorders and arthritis, may be improved through adding CBD to your day-to-day health care routine.

CBD is what we call a cannabinoid. Cannabinoids are chemical compounds found in the cannabis and hemp plant. Within our bodies, they work in a similar way to compounds called endocannabinoids that our own bodies produce naturally. CBD is one of the most effective compounds to help support our immune system, decrease anxiety and depression as well as being an influential neuroprotectant, defending and supporting the vital neurons that make up our brain function. Two major contributors to the breakdown of brain cells are oxidation and inflammation – CBD has very robust antioxidant and anti-inflammatory properties.

In addition to being an antioxidant and anti-inflammatory, CBD possesses an impressive assortment of therapeutic

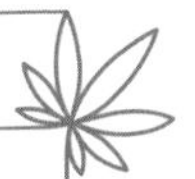

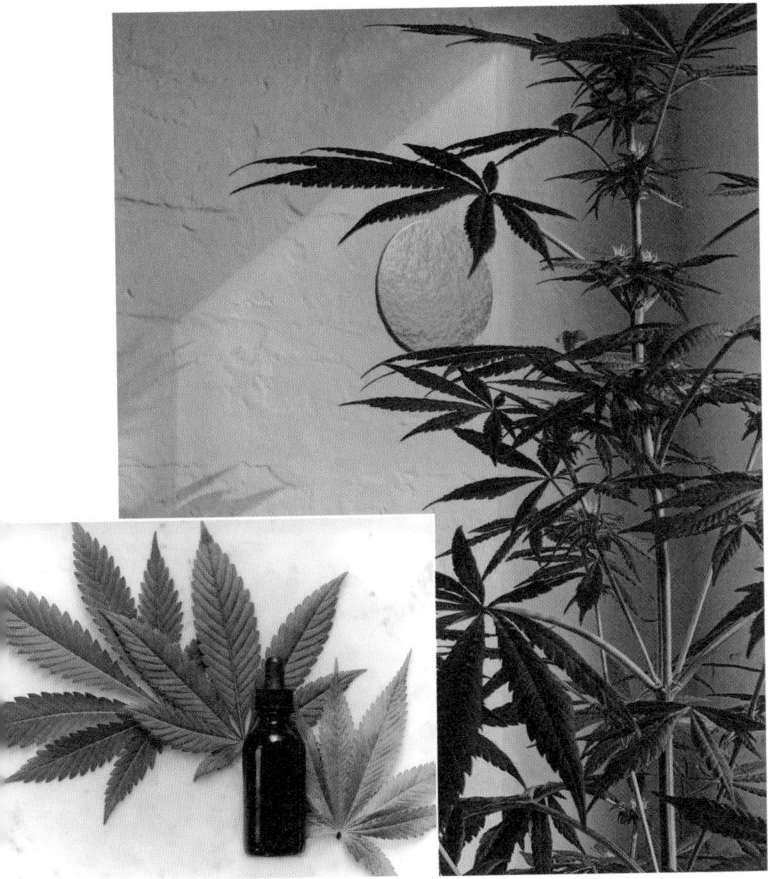

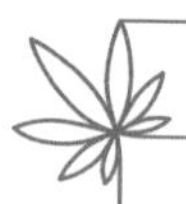

properties including anticonvulsant, anti-anxiety, analgesic, and antidepressant, as well as having neuroprotective capabilities. CBD is the non-psychoactive component of cannabis and hemp and cannabis plant. Many of these properties are enormously advantageous when treating skin conditions, including dehydration, dullness, blotchiness, acne, psoriasis, eczema and uneven pigmentation. However, CBD reaches far beyond the epidermal layers of our skin on her therapeutic journey. (CBD is always made from female plants so the pronoun is appropriate.)

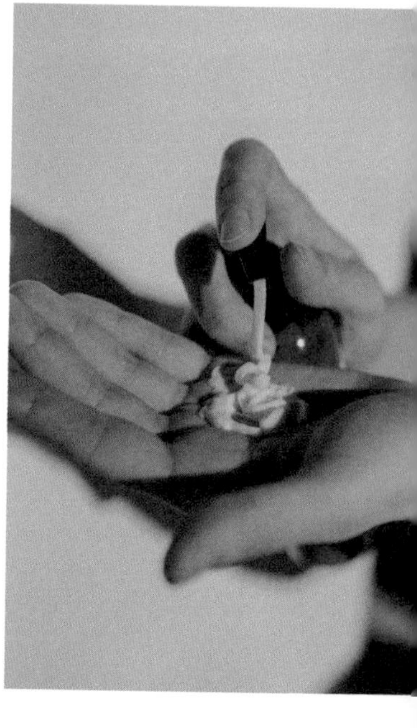

Initially CBD was recognized for her ability to reduce seizures and that became her original claim to fame. We now know, however — based on research and anecdotally — that CBD can also reduce pain, inflammation, arthritis, muscle spasms as well as helping to stimulate bone growth and help reduce blood sugar levels, which helps to control diabetes.

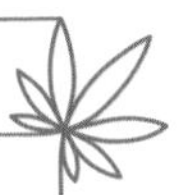

CBD is being successfully used to treat various health concerns, but the sturdiest scientific evidence is for her effectiveness in treating some of the harshest childhood epilepsy syndromes, such as Dravet syndrome and Lennox-Gastaut syndrome. Classically, these types of epilepsy do not respond effectively to pharmaceutical antiseizure medications. CBD on the other hand is able to reduce the number of seizures, and in some cases stop them altogether. In the US, the first FDA approved CBD-derived medicine, Epidiolex, is designed and used to treat the symptoms of these epilepsy syndromes.

She has also been found to be effective in the treatment of anxiety, insomnia, chronic pain and addiction. CBD is proving useful both to help us fall asleep and to stay asleep. With addiction, she helps to lower tobacco and heroin cravings and is being widely used to tackle the opioid crisis in North America by helping to wean patients off their addictive opioid medication while also alleviating the pain they are suffering. Medically, CBD is being used most effectively for inflammatory and neuropathic pain.

Are you fascinated by this formidable natural compound yet? Wait until you meet the endocannabinoid system! The science behind CBD is remarkable, but once you understand how she works inside our body, CBD becomes justifiably captivating.

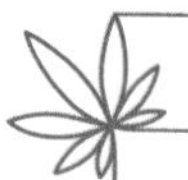

What is our endocannabinoid system?

Our physical wellbeing relies on an ever-shifting balance, a physiological juggling act performed by our bodies, called homeostasis. This process ensures that enzymes, the catalysts for the biochemical reactions that are constantly occurring within us, can function properly without disruption. When this balance is lost, the systems that keep us healthy can begin to collapse, which can result in some pretty undesirable health concerns.

In order to maintain homeostasis, the body utilizes a complex cell-signalling process known as the endocannabinoid system (ECS). Our bodies naturally create endocannabinoid molecules, neurotransmitters which bind to receptors in our central and peripheral nervous systems when homeostasis is disrupted by illness, injury or emotional distress. The ECS — comprised of endocannabinoids and the receptors in the body they bond with, and the enzymes that break these cannabinoids down — is like a safety net under the balancing act, giving our bodies the security needed to regain their balance and resume optimal activity.

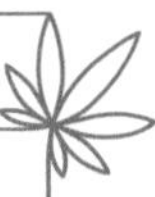

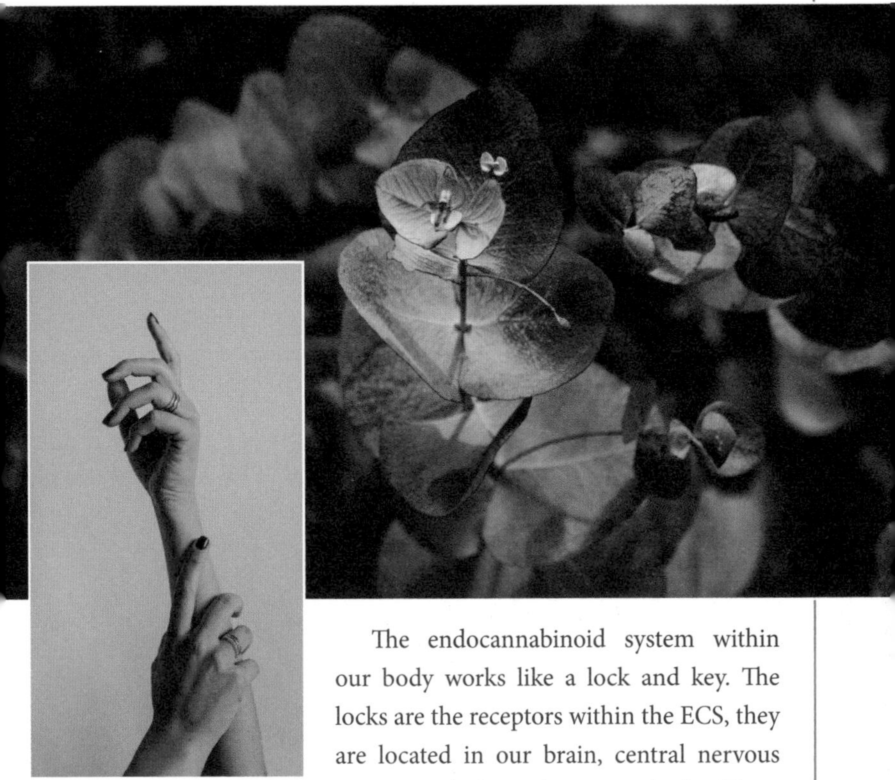

The endocannabinoid system within our body works like a lock and key. The locks are the receptors within the ECS, they are located in our brain, central nervous system and throughout our body. These receptors are called CB1 and CB2. CBD is the key that unlocks these receptors feeding the ECS, consequently giving it the fuel

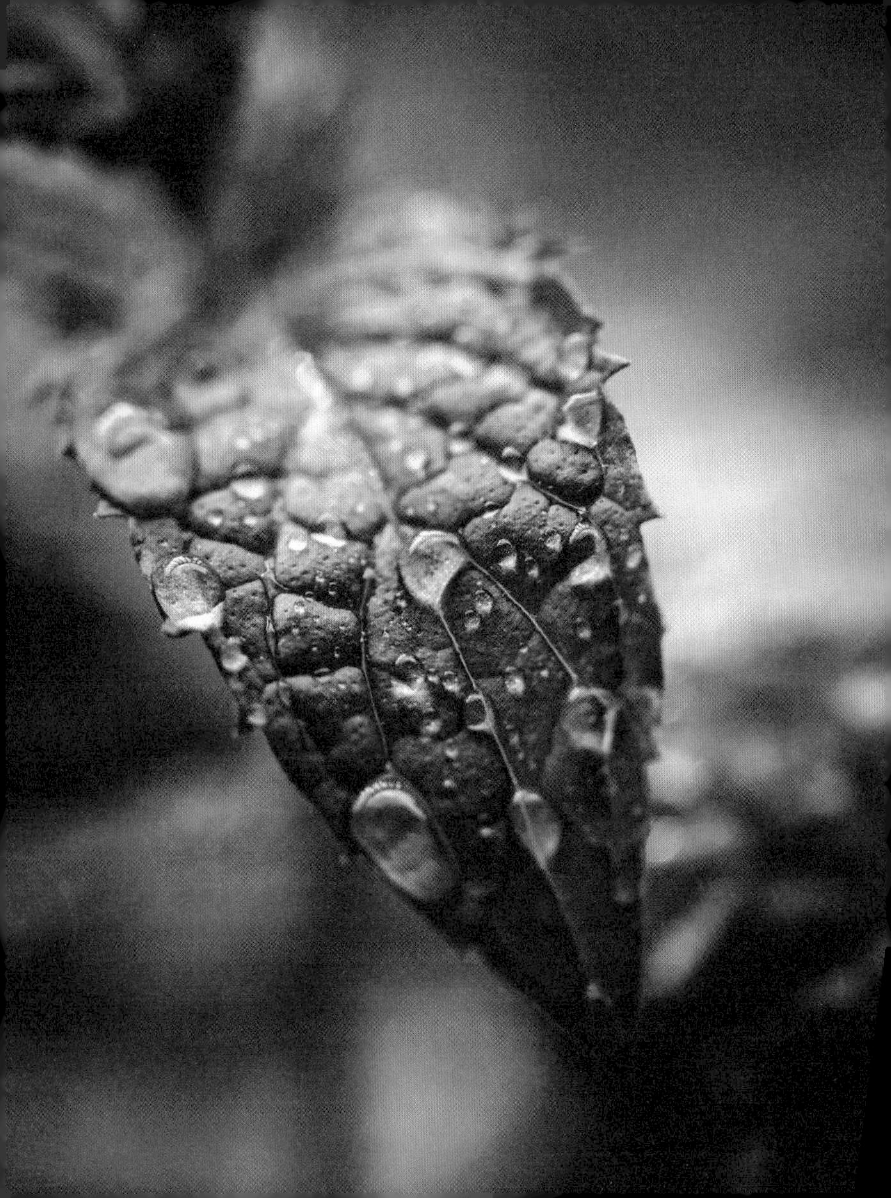

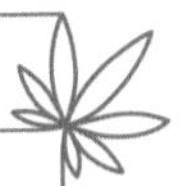

it needs to thrive for the betterment of our health. The endocannabinoid system is a remarkable network of compounds and receptors, often described as a central component of the health and healing of every human. This vast system has the capacity to influence functions in the brain, including memory, mood, pain response, appetite, perception, cognition, sleep, emotions, motor function and anti- inflammatory function as well as brain development and protection.

The endocannabinoid system is ubiquitous in the body —in the skin, the brain, major organs, connective tissue, glands, immune cells, etc. In each area of the body it carries out different tasks but the goal is always the same. It is a rather wonderful one: the ECS works tirelessly to maintain the body's internal balance and physical wellbeing. It creates an internal equilibrium, harmony and peace that resists even the most hostile fluctuations in the external environment.

It is amazing to think we have this system within our body, working every day to protect us and we didn't even know about it officially until the early 90s. In 1988, in a government-funded study at the St Louis University School of Medicine, Allyn Howlett and William Devane determined that the brains of mammals have receptor sites that respond to compounds found in cannabis. These receptors, named cannabinoid receptors,

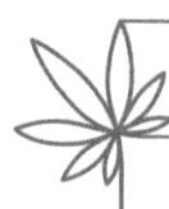

turned out to be the most abundant type of neurotransmitter receptor in the brain. It was not until 1992, however, that the endocannabinoid system was discovered by Dr Raphael Mechoulam of the Hebrew University of Jerusalem, who was researching the cannabis plant at the time. It is almost unbelievable to think this discovery is just under 30 years old, considering that the ECS is so fundamentally important.

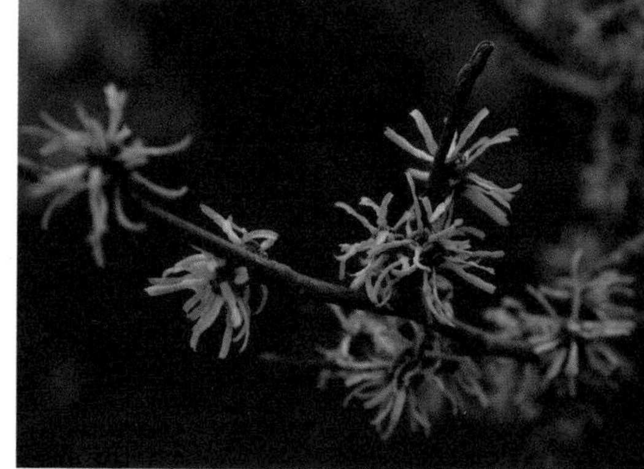

As Italian researcher, Vincenzo Di Marzo, says, the ECS is "essential to life's basic processes by relaying messages that affect how we relax, eat, sleep, forget and protect."

The endocannabinoid system is fed by two types of cannabinoids: phytocannabinoids (also known as plant cannabinoids) and endocannabinoids (also called endogenous cannabinoids – cannabinoids produced naturally in the body). These two types of cannabinoids are so incredibly similar that our body responds

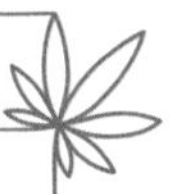

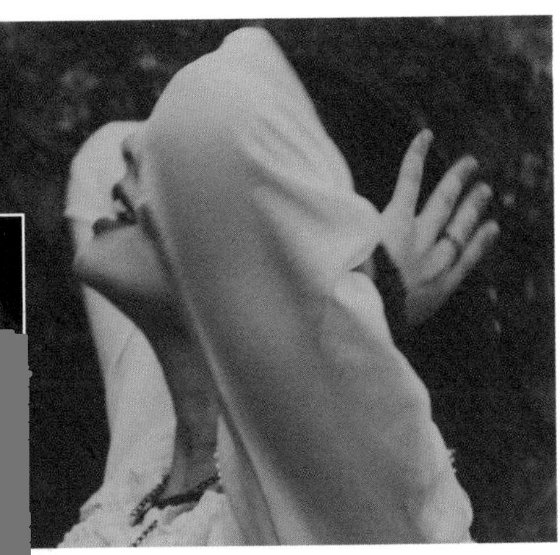

to them as though they are one and the same. At times when our body, on its own, does not produce enough endocannabinoids to maintain that desirable state of homeostasis, it will happily use phytocannabinoids to make up the shortfall.

It is safe to say the endocannabinoid system is the controlling system of fundamentally all functions within our body and mind, and CBD feeds our endocannabinoid system.

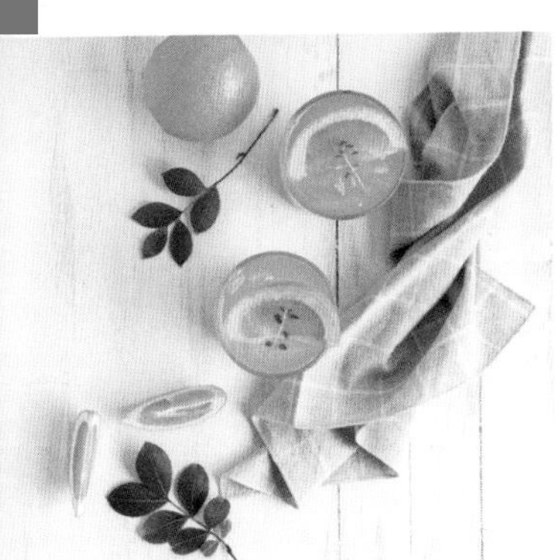

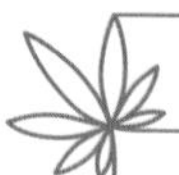

What happens when we don't feed the endocannabinoid system?

There is a body of scientific evidence that says if our ENC is not fed and optimized, we will suffer from that is called clinical endocannabinoid deficiency (CECD). The theory behind this syndrome is that, because our body only produces endocannabinoids on demand, our ECS benefits when we supplement these with phytocannabinoids. If we do not produce enough cannabinoids, we will suffer from clinical endocannabinoid deficiency.

Dr Ethan Russo is one of the leading scientific experts in the field of endocannabinoid science, and his work has focused on clinical endocannabinoid deficiencies, which he describes as impacting negatively on digestion, mood, anxiety, sleep, pain, and inflammation. He says that EDS is also associated with migraines, fibromyalgia and irritable bowel syndrome.

For the last two decades, the theory of clinical endocannabinoid deficiency has been studied and it is now connected to

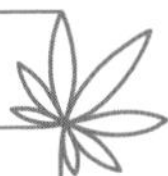

some specific illnesses. Animal studies have been carried out to test the efficiency of cannabinoids. In the studies, clinical endocannabinoid deficiency was mimicked by deleting the CB1 and CB2 receptors. The results have shown that a few conditions are relevant to the deficit when this happens, namely Alzheimer's, diabetes, stress, anxiety conditions, inflammation and heart disease. It has also been discovered that reduced levels of anandamide and 2-AG have been found in patients with post-traumatic stress disorder (PTSD). This research is early and needs more clinical work.

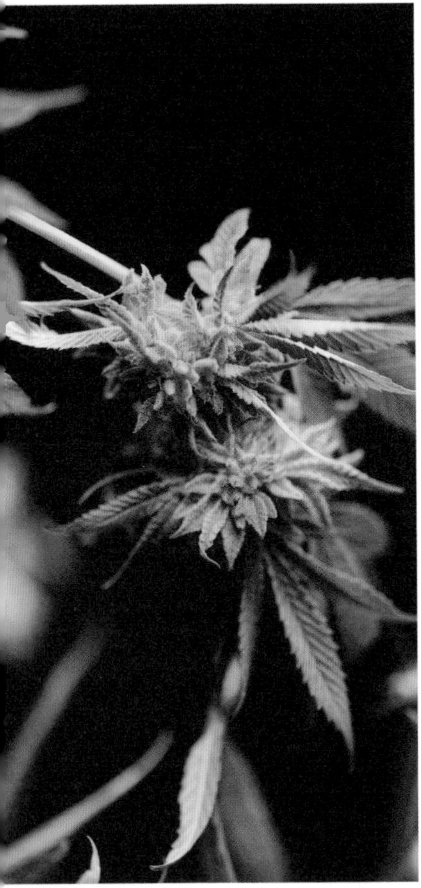

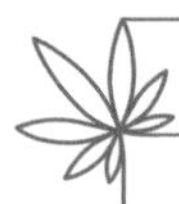

Understanding the plant

So, we now know CBD is a cannabinoid and we have encountered the endocannabinoid system, but what about the plant? Is hemp and cannabis the same thing or totally different? What is weed and is CBD even legal? Let me explain!

Every plant has a botanical name as well as a common name. Cannabis sativa is the botanical name for both the cannabis and the hemp plants. Both cannabis and hemp are Cannabis sativas. Hemp is one of the oldest domesticated crops ever farmed. Throughout history, we have grown different varieties of sativa for various purposes including to make clothing, for fibrous building material, rope, sails, biofuel, plastic and food. Today, some hemp plants are grown predominantly for their fibre, while others are grown primarily for their seeds to produce vegetable oil, which is used commonly in beauty care and cooking.

The difference between cannabis and hemp is all in the plant chemistry, which makes up the DNA of each plant. Cannabis has a full array of cannabinoids whereas hemp contains all the cannabinoids, but its legal THC level is very low, always 0.3% or below. Pot, weed, marijuana and other quirky names for the plant are all slang terms.

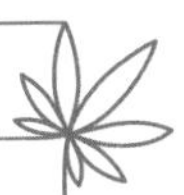

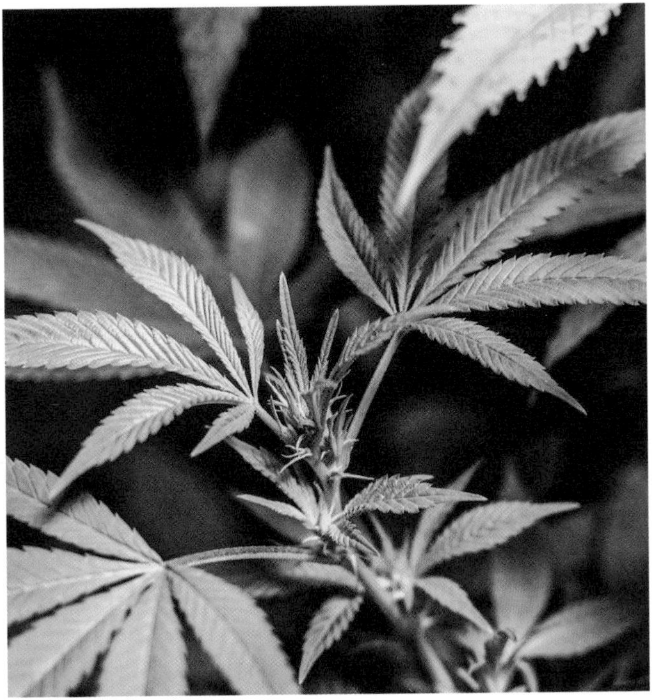

Cannabis sativa plants are also popular for medicinal and religious purposes, but unless cannabis is legal where you live, you will need a medical card, medical recommendation, or access to a legally approved dispensary in order to access

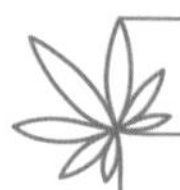

medical cannabis. Hemp is used mostly for its CBD content and contains low levels of THC; legally, it is the recommended plant of use. It is CBD from hemp that is used mostly within the beauty and cosmetic industry today. You can buy CBD oil extracted from hemp online, in beauty or health stores, and even in supermarkets.

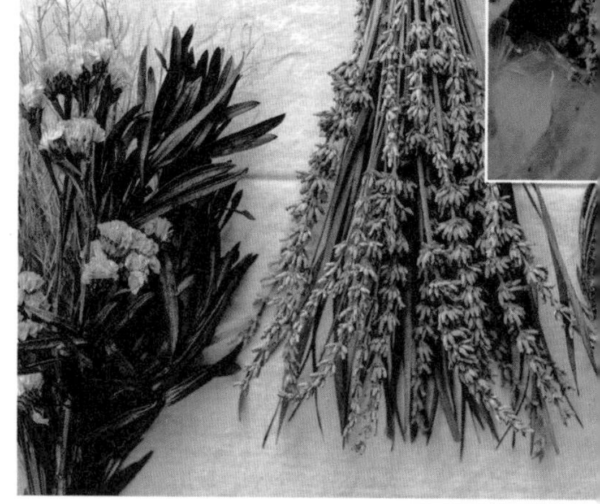

In the UK, CBD oil is always extracted from hemp, whereas in Canada and the USA CBD oil can be extracted from either hemp or cannabis. You need to read the label to understand which variety of the plant your CBD oil has come from. More on how to correctly and legally buy CBD later.

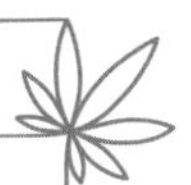

CBD Botany

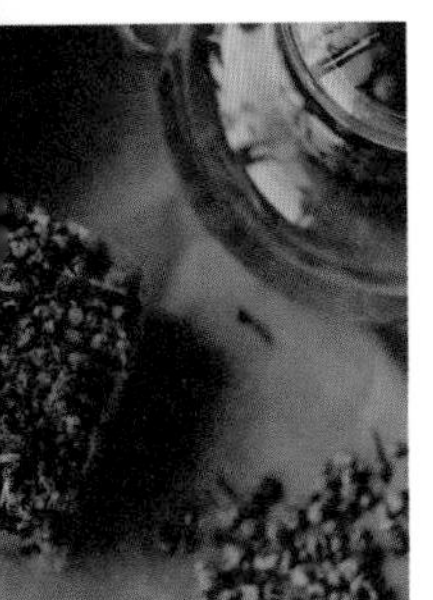

Cannabis plants vary in height from 3 to 15 feet tall and have numerous branches with five to seven delicate jagged leaves spread like fingers. The plant in its entirety is covered with tiny, sticky hair-like structures. These hairs are microscopic gland-like spikes that develop on the plant's skin. The technical term for these plant hairs is trichomes.

Trichomes are living cells. They serve to protect the leaves and flowers, and help reduce evaporation by protecting the plant from wind and heat. These trichomes contain an oily resin which is packed with the beneficial phytocannabinoids that make the cannabis plant so valuable to our health and skincare.

Cannabis has two main species, cannabis sativa and cannabis indica. While they are both versions of the same plant, their properties are quite different. Cannabis sativa produces more CBD and less than 1% THC; whereas cannabis indica is the drug-rich cannabis whose THC levels can be between 1% and 30%. Cannabis indica is the species that will get you high!

Depending on where and how the plant is grown, the phytochemical composition of these trichomes changes and each

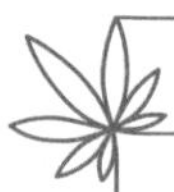

strain will have a unique therapeutic effect.

The same trichomes that release the potent phytochemicals from the cannabis plant also release another treasure, the highly aromatic compounds called terpenes. These little gems are also found in most essential oils. They are responsible for the colour and aroma of both essential oils and cannabis, and will substantially influence the medicinal and psychoactive effects of the plant and its extracted oil.

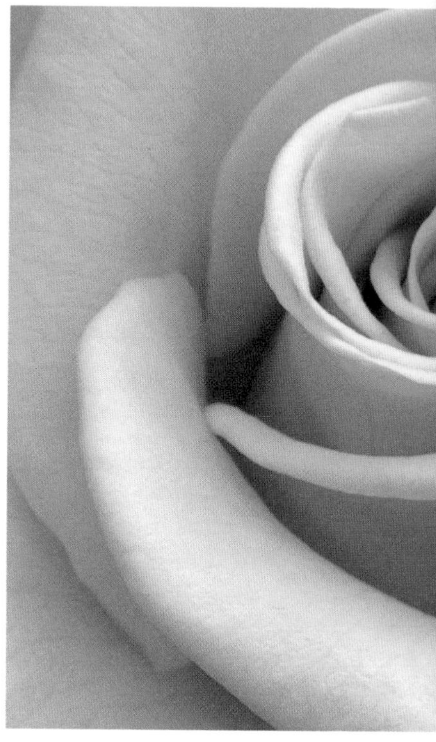

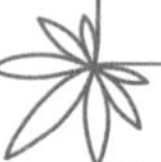

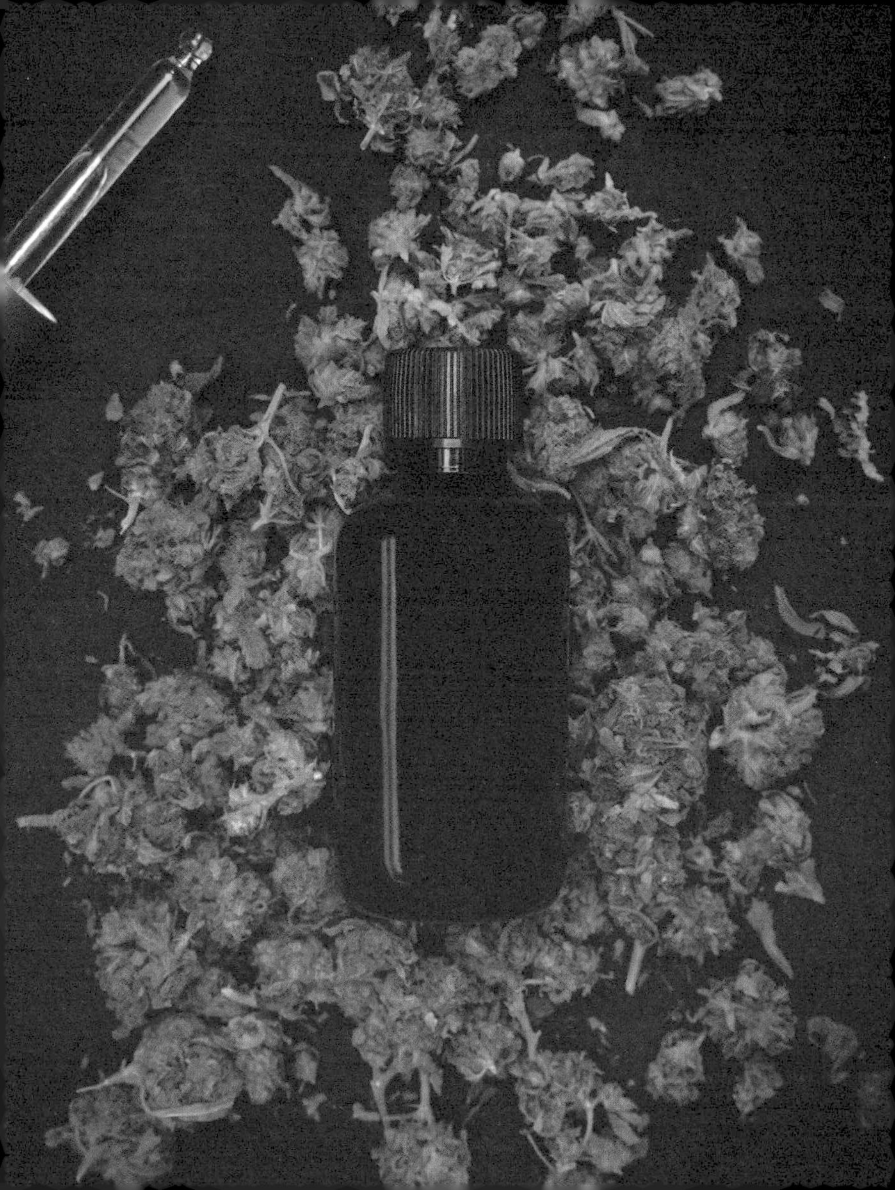

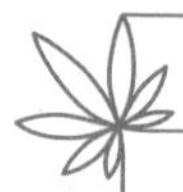

Tetrahydrocannabinol

I have mentioned a compound THC (Tetrahydrocannabinol) a few times now so let's take a breath and just get some clarity on this "controversial" compound.

THC, like CBD, is a cannabinoid found in the cannabis and, to a much lesser extent, hemp plants. THC can cause psychoactive effects depending on dosage and previous exposure to the cannabinoid. However, it is also an impressive therapeutic compound which is being effectively used to treat a wide range of medical conditions and symptoms including: pain relief, nausea, muscle spasms, appetite stimulation, anxiety, depression, and post-traumatic stress disorder (PTSD). Specifically, THC helps nauseous and sick patients to regain their appetite. Even patients

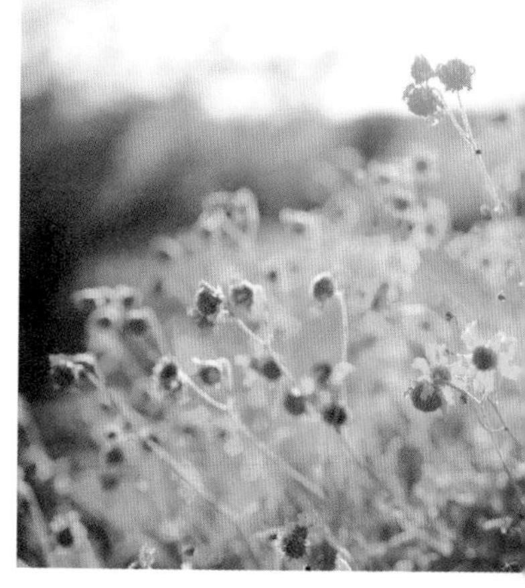

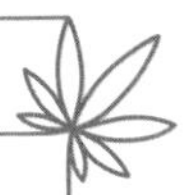

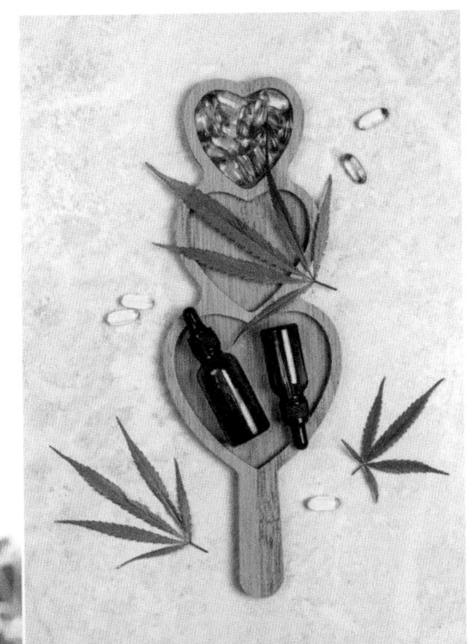

who suffer from cancer and debilitating pain have seen effective results medicating with THC. This is very encouraging, given the potential for addiction when treating with other forms of analgesia-like opioids. The medicinal applications for THC are undeniable and, as a result, pharmaceutical companies are now creating synthetic versions of THC to treat patients who suffer from the aforementioned conditions. So, THC and CBD may be sister compounds but they are very different in their impact on our body and mind.

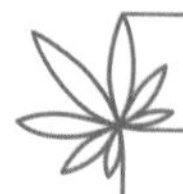

Plant Materials

A cannabis and hemp material is a material – whether liquid, solid or powder – which has been derived from the cannabis or hemp plant. These materials can be derived from the whole plant or an isolated part of the plant.

There are more and more cannabis and hemp materials available to us today, but this area can be a minefield. You will need to decide which materials best suit your particular requirements, taking into account the legal environment where you live. Here we will look at how cannabinoids are extracted from the plant and what CBD materials are available to us.

Cannabis and hemp plants are most typically extracted by a process called CO_2 extraction, or supercritical CO_2 extraction. This extraction method uses a chemical solvent such as ethanol, propane, butane or hexane. The solvents are used to dissolve the plant into a solution or crude. The crude is then distilled in order to isolate certain components from the plant: phytocannabinoids, terpenes, flavonoids, chlorophyll and even waxes can be extracted through chemical extraction methods. This produces concentrates (also known as extracts). Once the extraction is complete, the solvents need to be purged from the resinous oil.

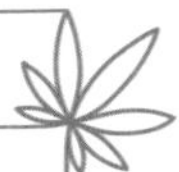

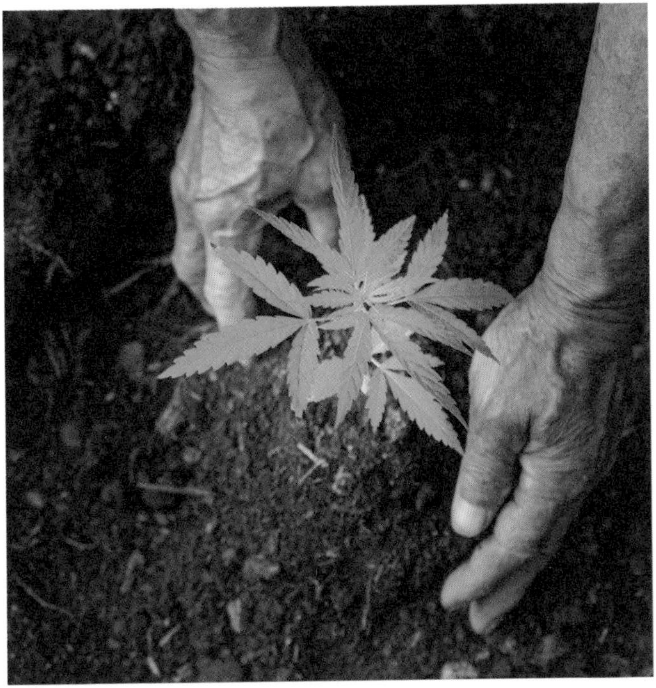

This can be achieved by employing evaporation, vacuuming or hand-whipping. The aim is to remove the residual solvent from the extracted material to give us a clean cannabinoid-rich material.

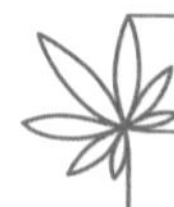

THE THREE MAIN MATERIALS YOU CAN PURCHASE ARE EXPLAINED HERE:

Full Spectrum

Full spectrum material, also known as whole plant material, is a direct extract from the raw cannabis or hemp plants. It contains the full range of phytocannabinoids, terpenes, flavonoids, fatty acids and other phytochemicals. While this can vary according to the strain of the plant from which the material is extracted, full spectrum extract tends to have higher levels of phytocannabinoids and, in most cases, deliberately cultivated high levels of either THC or CBD – or even both. Full spectrum extract is most commonly used in medicinal and recreational products. Full spectrum naturally contains terpenes which amplify the effect of phytocannabinoids when interacting with the endocannabinoid system.

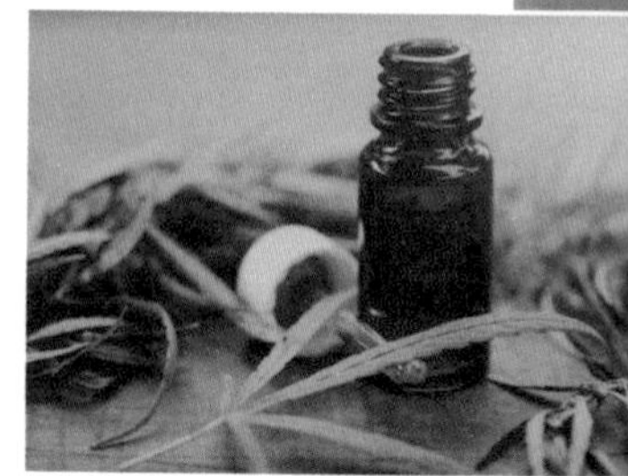

Distillate

Distillate is also known as broad spectrum CBD, or CBD distillate. It is an extract which retains all the phytocannabinoids, terpenes, flavonoids, fatty acids, and phytochemicals of the

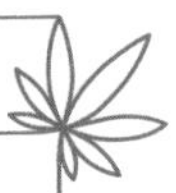

original plant. This extract then goes through a special process after extraction to remove the THC cannabinoid. While this can vary according to the strain of the plant from which the material is extracted, distillate tends to have high levels of CBD as well as a range of other naturally occurring cannabinoids. Distillate is considered ideal for people who want to experience the benefits of full-spectrum without the THC content. It is used a lot in skincare and herbal products where brands or medicine makers don't want to take the risk of accidentally using illegal levels of THC. Distillate naturally contains terpenes, which amplify the effect of phytocannabinoids when interacting with the endocannabinoid system.

Isolate

CBD isolate is CBD in its purest form. During the extraction process, all phytochemicals are removed or filtered out of the cannabis or hemp plant except for the CBD. Typically, a CBD isolate is between 90–97% isolate. The higher the percentage of CBD the better.

Isolate is used in medicinal and recreational product preparations but not as frequently as full-spectrum and distillate. It is used a lot in beauty products, since there is no risk of violating the THC legal limitation of 0.3%.

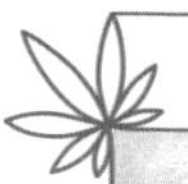

WHAT CBD IS NOT

One thing CBD will not do is get you high. It can relax you and ease anxiety, but it will not produce the impaired psychotropic effect which the cannabinoid THC provides. CBD and THC should not be confused with each other. CBD is the second most predominant active ingredient in the cannabis plant, only second to its sister cannabinoid, THC.

Hemp Essential Oil

You may see a product called cannabis or hemp essential oil; it is important to understand that this admittedly lovely oil is not CBD oil. An "essential oil" is a distillation of plant material and this action captures the volatile components, for example the aromatic terpenes. Cannabinoids are considered non-volatiles; they are fat loving, not water loving. This means that they cannot be distilled effectively and therefore cannot end up in the plant's essential oil.

Hemp Seed Oil

Many people buy hempseed oil under the illusion that it is CBD oil - it is not. Hempseed oil is produced by pressing hempseeds, which do NOT contain phytocannabinoids. Let me be super clear here: hempseed oil does not have any CBD in there — not even a token dose!

However, hempseed oil is a wonderful vegetable oil for skincare recipes. It is stunningly therapeutic, rich in vitamin E and holds a treasure trove of essential fatty acids which make it a restorative, regenerative, replenishing, anti-inflammatory and antioxidant skincare ingredient. It has the ability to protect and repair the skin from cellular damage while soothing irritation and balancing sebum production.

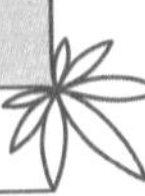

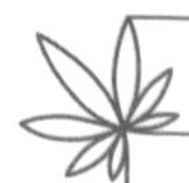

Taking CBD

CBD can be consumed in many forms, including oils, extracts, capsules, patches, vapes, and topical preparations for use on skin. Depending on why you are using CBD you will choose the delivery route and product best suited to tackle that problem. For example, if you are aiming to decrease inflammation and relieve muscle and joint pain, a topical CBD-infused oil, lotion or cream is the best choice. We know that topical CBD products interact with cannabinoid receptors in the skin and nervous system. Applying CBD oil to the skin is one of the most efficacious ways to use the compound when consistently applied directly to areas of chronic inflammation or pain, and if combined synergistically with other botanicals and essential oils to increase permeability. On the other hand, to successfully allow CBD to directly enter the bloodstream, a CBD tincture designed to be placed under the tongue is the best route of application.

CBD DOSAGE

CBD is most effective when taken every day. It is recommended to take 4–5 drops of high strength CBD oil, up to three times a

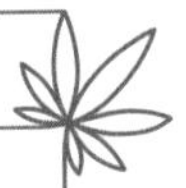

day. Take a moment and hold the drops under the tongue for 60 seconds before swallowing or in your coffee/hot drink is a great way to take your daily CBD dosage.

It is recommended to not exceed 80mg per day. A 10% strength CBD oil will provide 5mg of CBD per drop approximately. We are all different, so our bodies respond differently to CBD. When taken regularly, you may feel the positive impact of taking CBD instantly and for others it can take longer.

IS CBD SAFE?

You cannot overdose on CBD as such, but some people can experience mild side effects of CBD, for example nausea, fatigue, lack of focus and irritability. CBD can increase the level of blood thinning and other medicines in your blood by competing for the liver enzymes that break down these drugs. It is important to consult your doctor if you are under their care, taking life dependant medications or if you have health concerns before taking CBD.

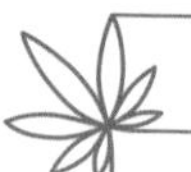

Buying CBD

There are so many CBD products on the market that you can accidently buy something that isn't proper CBD. There are some really quick and simple tips below to help you when purchasing CBD.

* **Legal considerations:** be sure you are familiar with the cannabis legislation where you live - don't buy cannabis where it is not legal.

* **Use a reputable brand:** when buying your CBD oil, it is important to choose reputable brands with a history in supplying plant-based concentrations.

* **CBD content:** it may sound obvious, but you do need to check that the product you are purchasing actually contains CBD! A lot of stores are selling hempseed vegetable oil as cannabis or CBD oil, which it is not. Equally, beware of products labelled hempseed oil and hemp essential oil - they do not contain CBD.

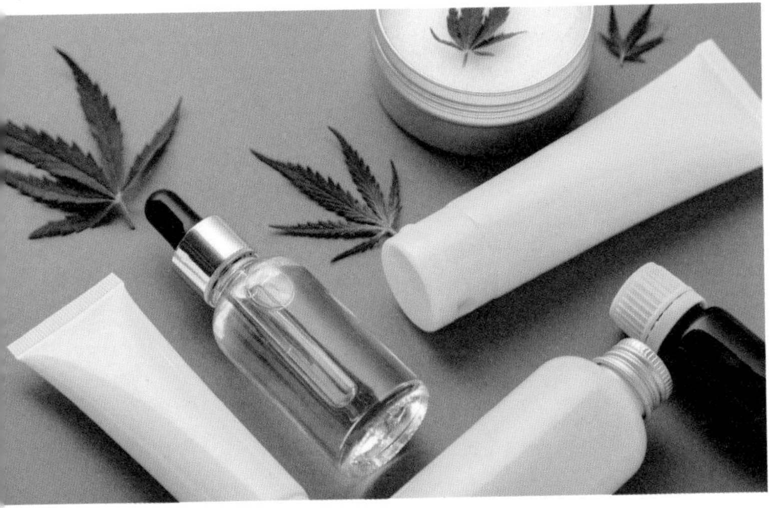

- **Look at the label!** It should have the following information:

    - **Concentration of CBD in your product.** While I have personally created products with up to 10,000mg of CBD oil per 30ml, I recommend a concentration of 300mg of CBD oil per 30ml for the recipes in this course.

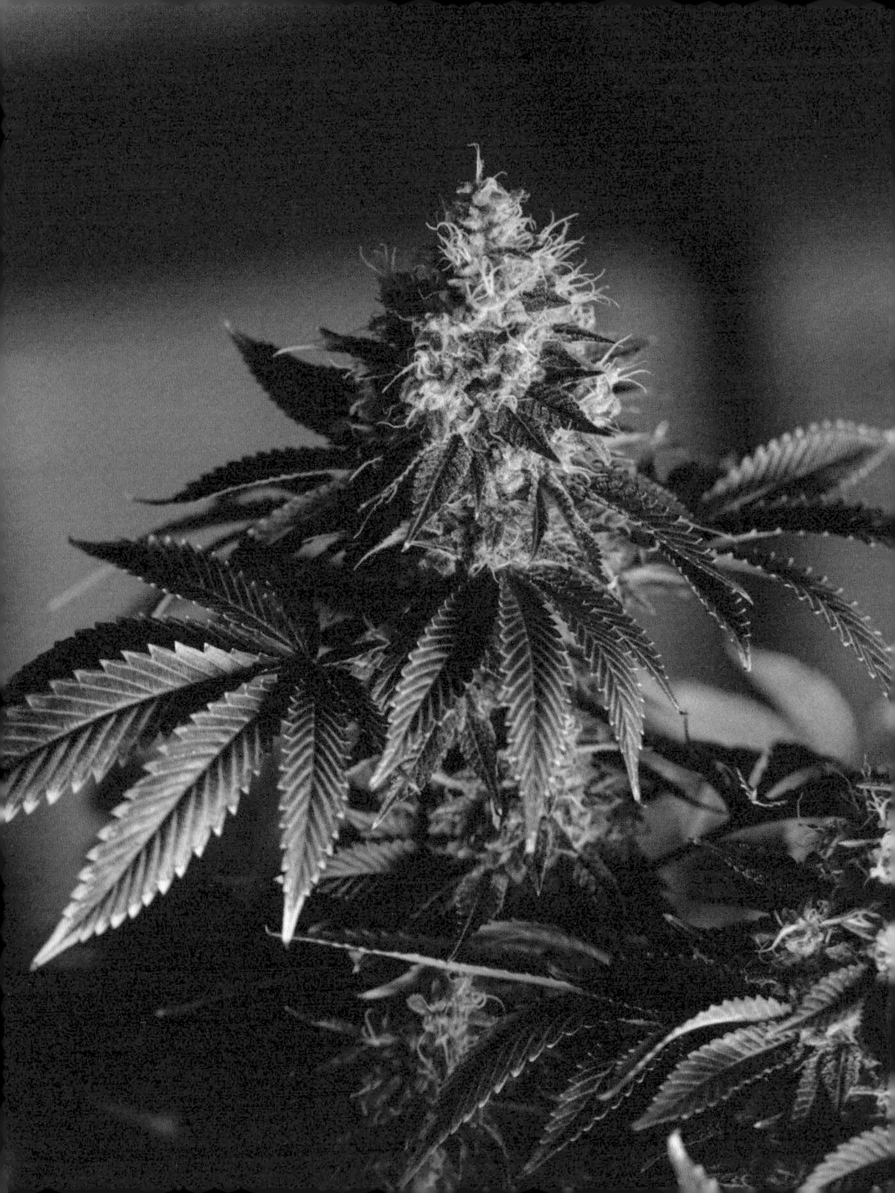

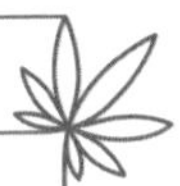

- **Batch number:** you need to see a batch number on the label to ensure the product is traceable to the manufacturer in case of any issues with it.

- **Best by date:** this is vital so you can gauge the freshness of the product and ensure you use it before it expires.

* **Lab report/Certificate of Analysis (COA):** It is very important to look for a Certificate of Analysis (COA) for the product you are interested in. This should be readily available on the brand's website. It is important to know if the analysis was performed by an accredited laboratory. A good indication will be if they are accredited in accordance with the International Organization for Standardization (ISO). This report will show you the CBD concentration. It is a nice comfort check to ensure your product truly has the CBD concentration advertised. Note that the lab report should be reasonably recent, preferably within the last 12 months.

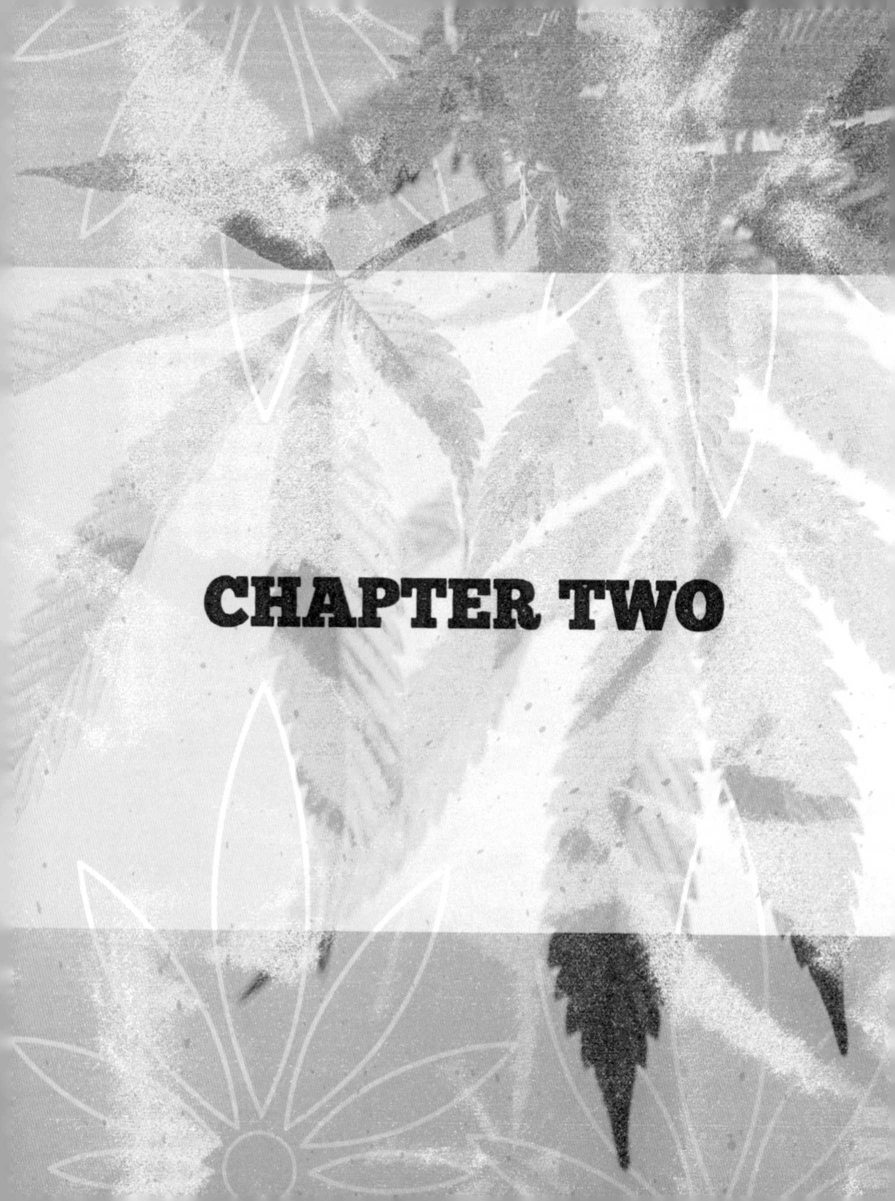

CHAPTER TWO

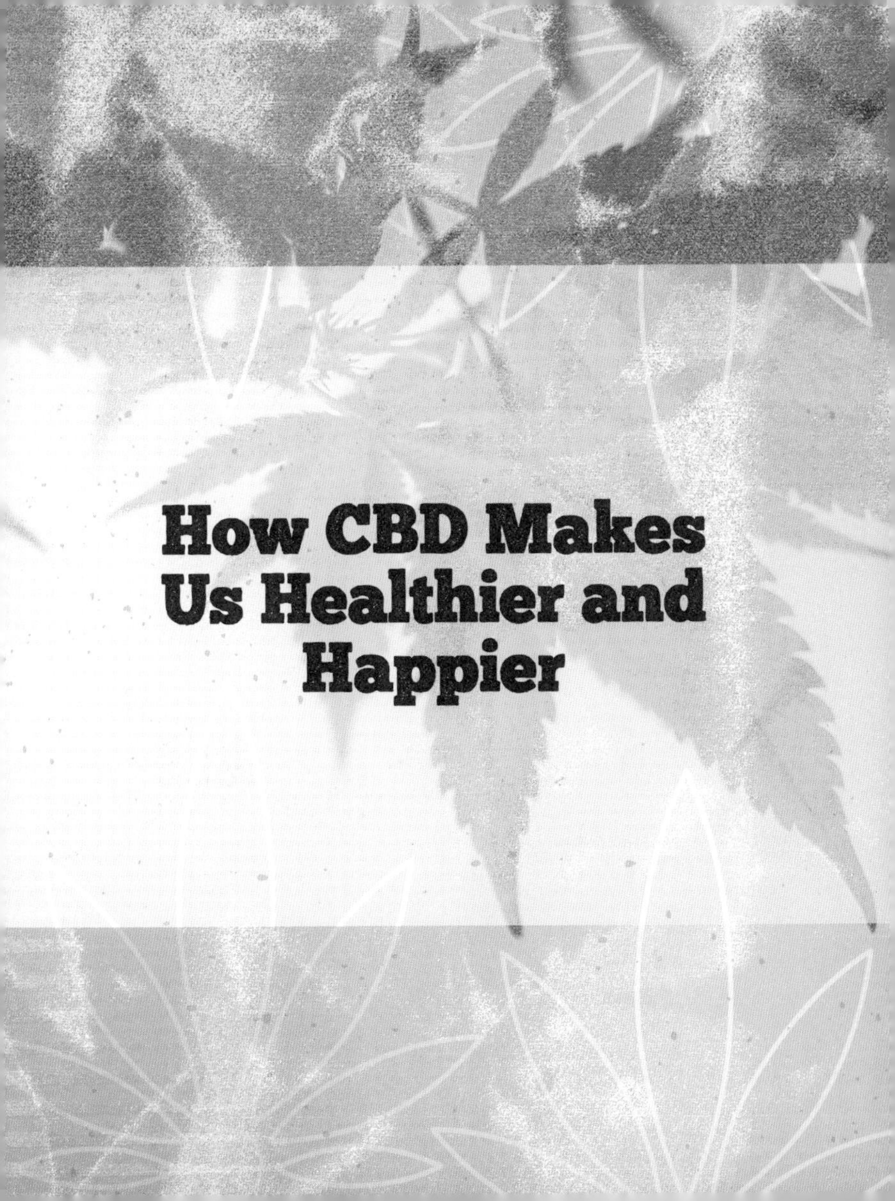

How CBD Makes Us Healthier and Happier

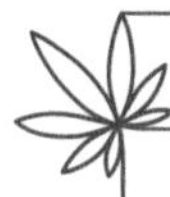

How can CBD enhance my day-to-day life?

There are common challenges we face every day from stress and anxiety, pain and sleep deprivation which affect how well we function in our daily lives. Stress and overwhelm have become so "normal", we accept them as part of daily life. They don't have to be. Stress-relieving CBD taken each day will lift the weight of overwhelm and relieve the pressure of stress.

It is important to note that some stress is good. It keeps us sharp, focused and safe. Stress is a human protection tool, but too much of it will deplete our immune system and fry our nervous system. How do we find the sweet stress spot? CBD will help regulate our stress levels and reactions. Add CBD to your daily health supplement routine and relieve the pressures of anxiety and overwhelm.

Add CBD to your daily health supplement routine and watch the weight of stress and overwhelm melt away to a distant memory.

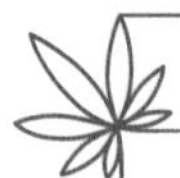

What is stress?

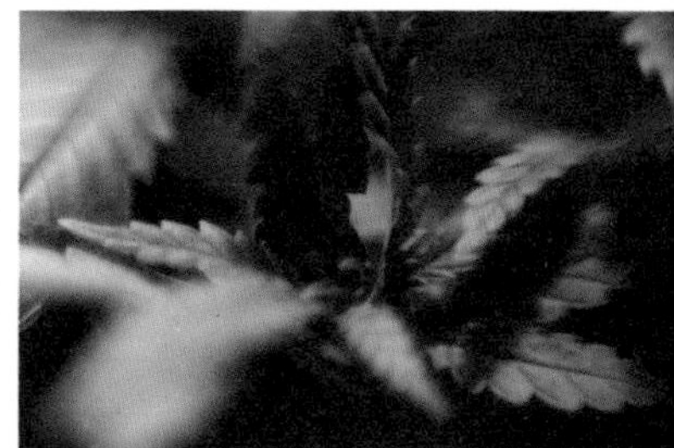

In Aesop's fable "The Town Mouse and the Country Mouse", the latter mouse hurriedly flees a luxurious but chaotic dinner at the former's home, exclaiming, "A crust eaten in peace is better than a banquet partaken in anxiety!" Some of us mice may be lucky enough to have a bolt-hole in the country to escape to, or a home by the sea, when the stresses and strains of modern life become too much. But stress, defined by Webster's dictionary as "a state resulting from a stress: one of bodily or mental tension resulting from factors that tend to alter an existent equilibrium", doesn't always stay where we left it. It follows us, lives inside us, invites itself to our table — wherever we may be.

Stress is both a physical and emotional phenomenon: the "fight or flight" hormones, adrenaline and cortisol, are released into the body when we feel anxious, raising our heart rate and causing rapid, shallow breathing. These physiological

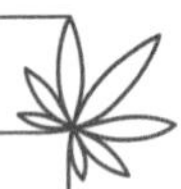

responses are helpful when we are faced with a genuine threat — more oxygen in the blood means an enhanced physical response. But when these changes in our body last significantly longer than the appropriate window of reaction to danger, they can lead to a variety of distressing outcomes such as stomach complaints, headaches, insomnia and depression. In many of us, anxiety can become a burdensome long-term condition, rather than a short-lived survival mechanism.

The American Journal of Managed Care estimates the annual cost of anxiety disorders to be between $42.3 billion and $46.6 billion, "of which more than 75% can be attributed to morbidity, mortality, lost productivity, and other indirect costs." Unmanaged anxiety is as expensive to the state as it is miserable to the sufferer. As St Augustine wrote in the Confessions: "The punishment of every disordered mind is its own disorder."

STRESS & HORMONES

Stress is bad for our blood pressure, mental state, and overall health. Cortisol, along with adrenaline, is involved in managing our stress response. Cortisol is a hormone produced in the adrenal gland that helps

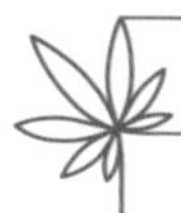

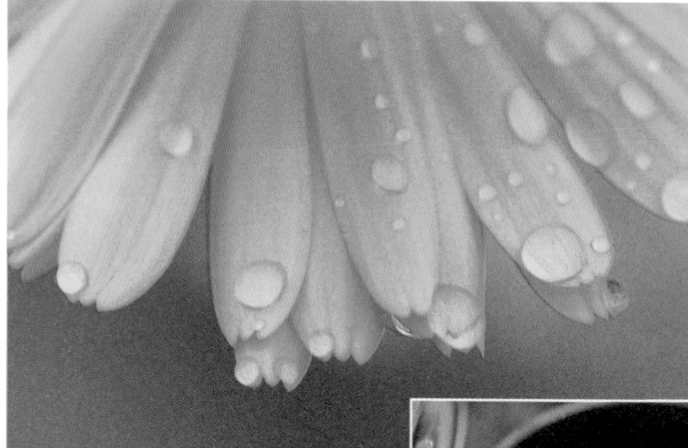

regulate blood sugar, metabolism, inflammation and memory formation. Most commonly referred to as the "stress hormone", cortisol is released during times of stress or crisis and, as a result, temporarily shuts down your digestion and reproduction systems. Cortisol is essential for survival. It's responsible for controlling our natural "flight or fight" response. If you produce too much cortisol, you may suffer symptoms,

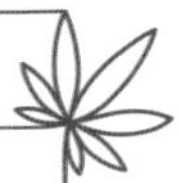

including weight gain, mood swings, and increased anxiety. CBD is able to lower cortisol levels, this hormone associated with chronic stress.

MANAGING STRESS AND ANXIETY WITH CBD

It is estimated about 40 million adults suffer from anxiety disorders in the United States. This includes generalized anxiety, social anxiety, panic and phobia disorders. CBD is being reported as a solution to help with anxiety. In 2018, the search term "CBD gummies" was the third most popular food-related Google search of the year.

Anxiety has accommodated us all through one life journey or another, and for some of us it is a constant presence in our daily lives. In recent years cannabis and CBD especially have stepped up as an effective, plant-based solution. But how does it work?

It all leads back to the endocannabinoid system. As you have learned, the primary function of the ECS is to maintain a balanced, neutral state called homeostasis. The ECS is believed to help modulate a wide range of physiological processes, including pain sensation, body temperature, memory, mood, appetite, stress, sleep, metabolism, immune function, and reproduction.

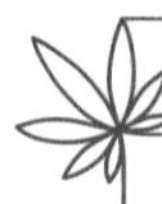

The ECS communicates through a class of compounds called endocannabinoids, which are messengers produced naturally by the body that attach to special receptors called CB1 and CB2. Cannabinoids like CBD found in the cannabis and hemp plant are similar to endocannabinoids. The cannabinoids have the ability to interact with these receptors. The ECS helps regulate function in many parts of the body, but when it comes to modulating stress and anxiety, it mostly works with the brain. There are circuits in our brain that are involved in generating shifts in behaviour states. The majority of this activity occurs in the part of the brain called the amygdala, which reacts to both real and perceived dangers, for example false alarms that trigger anxiety, by launching a fight-or-flight response — the heart beats faster, breathing speeds up, muscles tense, and an internal voice screams run!

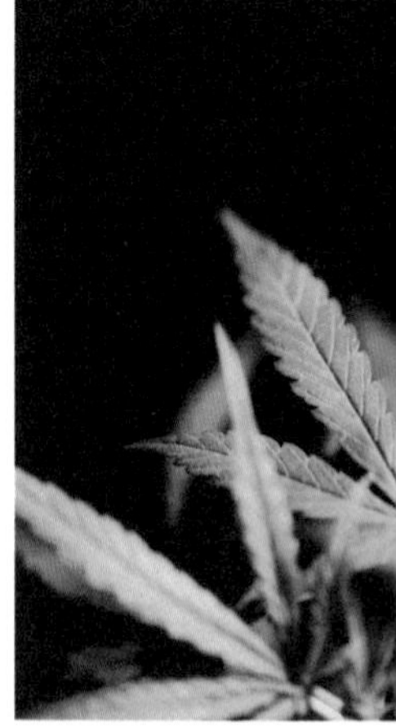

But the body has an override system: the ECS. Researchers have discovered that when the brain launches a stress response, the ECS can put on the brakes. It is known that endocannabinoids are involved in keeping the amygdala less active so that we don't produce stress or anxiety when there is no real danger or

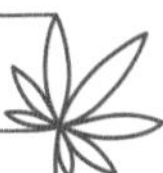

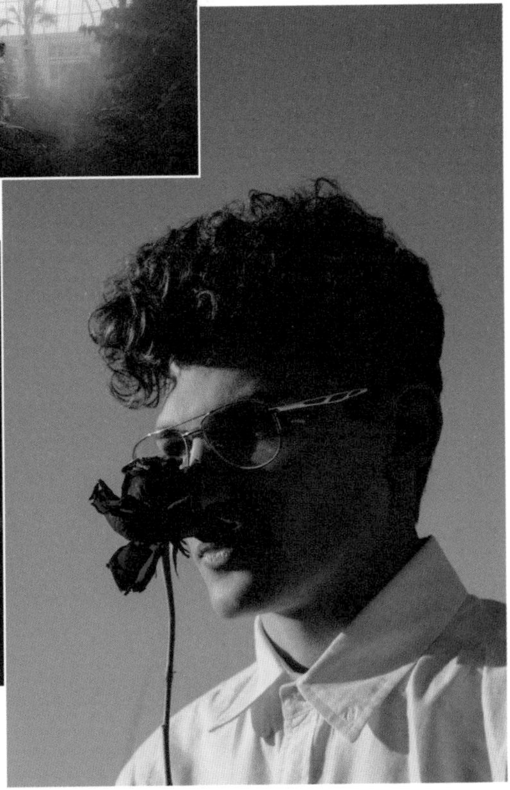

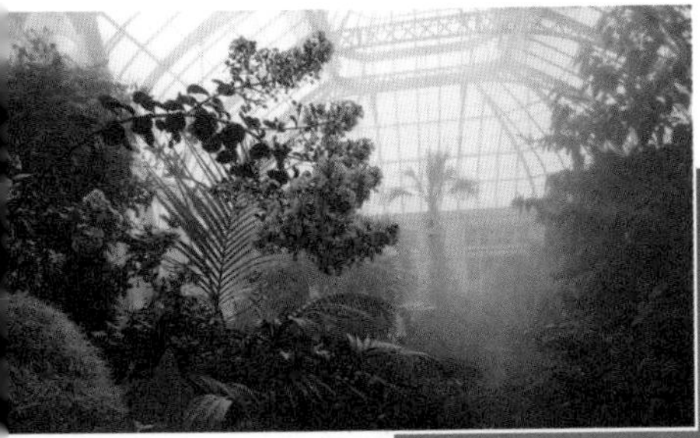

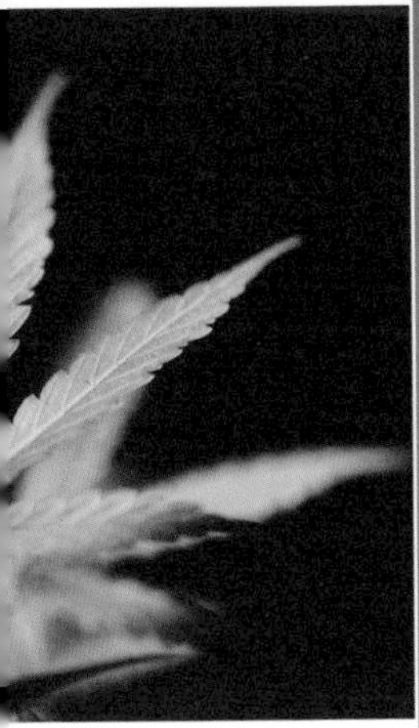

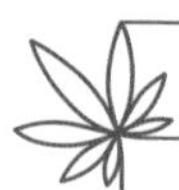

threat. But the ECS does not work on its own. By attaching to the CB1 receptor, endocannabinoids also help relay messages to other neurotransmitters involved in producing or preventing anxiety. This function is as vital, as researchers have learned that repeated exposure to stress can cause the ECS to burn out. This explains why habitually people under chronic stress are more vulnerable to stress-related mental-health conditions, such as anxiety.

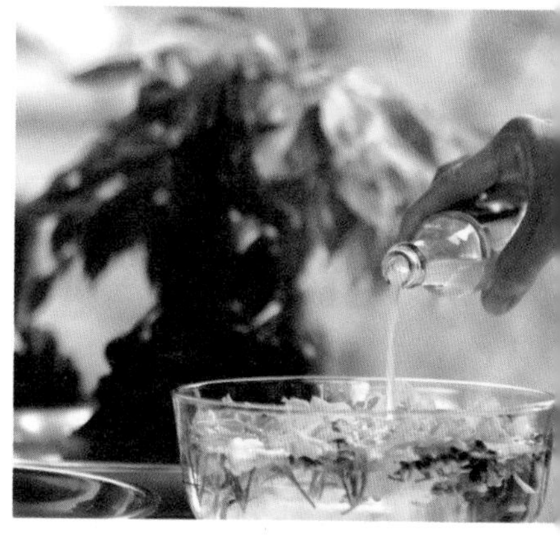

WHY IS CBD SO IMPORTANT IN THE STRESS AND ANXIETY CONVERSATION?

CBD interacts with the 5-HT1A and TRPV1 receptors, both of which help regulate fear and anxiety. In addition, the endocannabinoid system is known to be instrumental in mood regulation, plus a dysfunctional endocannabinoid system is associated with impaired fear-regulation. A systematic review of clinical CBD suggests that she can be effective at reducing generalized

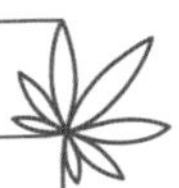

anxiety, social anxiety, panic disorder, obsessive compulsive disorder and post-traumatic stress disorder, and might mitigate THC-induced anxiety. A study published in 2019 which examined the efficacy of CBD for the treatment of anxiety and sleep disorders noted that dosages of CBD ranged from 25mg to 175mg/day. Anxiety sufferers responded better to the lower dosages and those with sleep disorders responded better to the higher dosages of CBD.

HOW CAN CBD HELP?

When we suffer from stress or anxiety, we ideally seek to manage its symptoms while working towards solutions to the challenges triggering our worries. In order to reach a feeling of equilibrium, where our real or perceived problems feel manageable again, we need the calm that comes from relaxation and restful sleep. CBD is known to promote calm, giving us access to the therapeutic tools that can lead to self-healing. But how does it work?

In order to maintain homeostasis, our internal state of physical equilibrium, the body uses a complex, cell-signalling process known as the endocannabinoid system. Our bodies naturally create endocannabinoid molecules, which bind to receptors in our central and peripheral nervous systems when

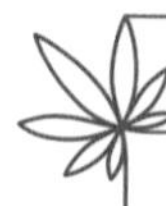

homeostasis is disrupted by illness, injury or emotional distress. Simply put, the ECS behaves like an emergency call-out service within us, responding to crises in the body whenever needed. CBD is believed to instead modify the receptors' ability to bind to cannabinoids, and also prevent them being broken down by enzymes in the body – allowing them to have longer-lasting beneficial effects, such as the feeling of wellness and serenity that results from a holistically-balanced mind, body and spirit. There is speculation in the scientific community that some people may also suffer from a condition called clinical endocannabinoid deficiency, for which CBD would seem to be a safe, logical and natural solution.

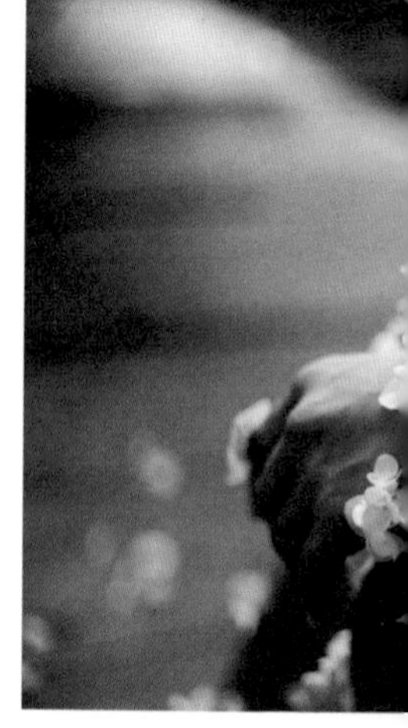

USING CBD OIL TO REDUCE STRESS AND ANXIETY

Ingesting CBD orally can provide long-lasting and systemic relief for anxiety that is moderate to severe, and which affects the patient's quality of life. Also, ingesting it consistently over a period of time can reduce inflammation and chronic anxiety and does not induce analgesic tolerance. Consider transdermal application such as a patch if the you require long-acting

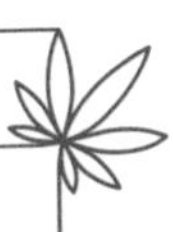

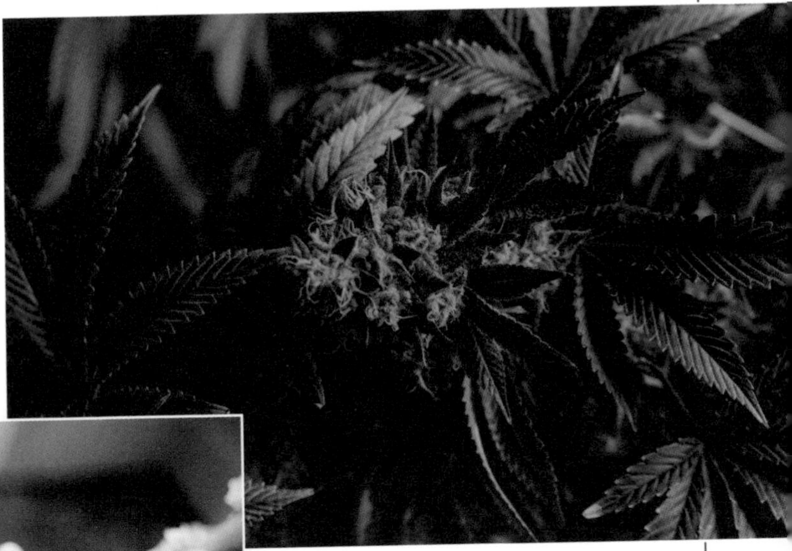

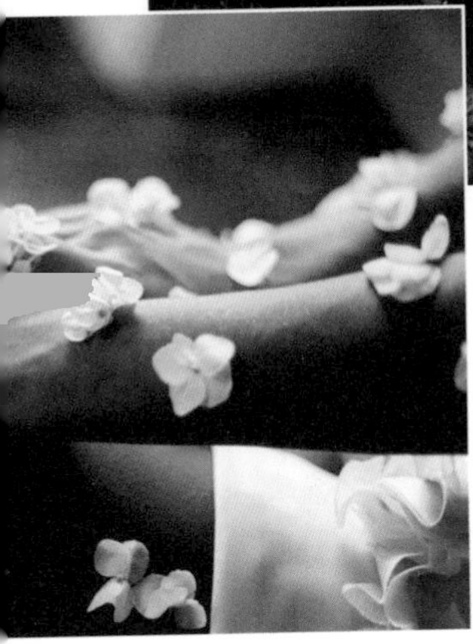

relief or cannot tolerate oral administration — maybe the taste is too much for you. Transdermal CBD patches can provide 8–12 hours of consistent cannabinoid release. Inhalation can be a good option for patients who suffer from panic attacks or extreme anxiety, as this route can quickly

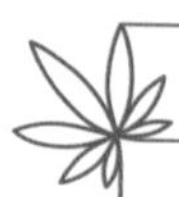

relieve anxiety and give patients the most control over their dose. For example, you can inhale CBD and experience potential relief within minutes. Topical products can also provide some relief from anxiety symptoms but not as much as some other methods as they don't work systemically. Also using CBD with essential oils in a topical product can be super effective!

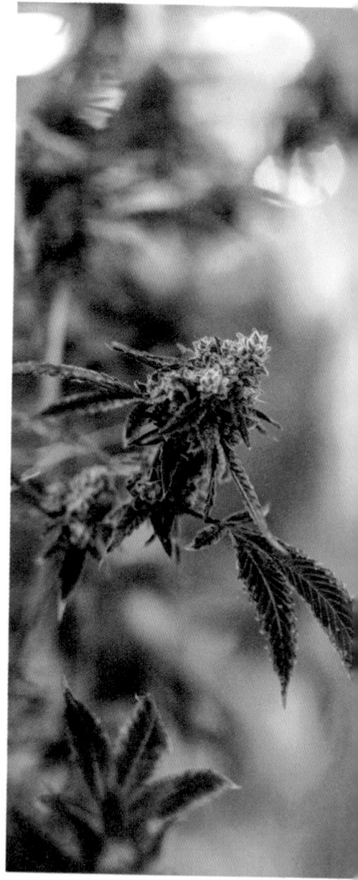

Research suggests that a low dose of 50 to 75mg of CBD oil a day can reduce anxiety and improve sleep quality within a month. It can be taken by mouth in oils and tinctures from dropper bottles, in chewable gummies, or in capsules, sprays or vapes. Unlike THC, CBD is understood to produce little if any side effects and is deemed safe by the World Health Organization.

It is worth thinking about the type of

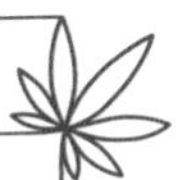

stress and anxiety you need relief from when considering these options. For example, vaping releases CBD into the bloodstream more quickly than the ingestion of oil or gummies, so may be the preferred method of consumption before anxiety-inducing scenarios such as public speaking or social interaction. When seeking restful sleep, or day-to-day calm and relaxation, ingestion may prove more appropriate. Start on low doses, and keep a journal of your body's response. While doses as high as 600mg of CBD a day have been proven efficacious in the treatment of post-traumatic disorder, for example, a much lower dose of as little as 25mg may be a sensible (and much less expensive) starting point.

You can escape that overwhelming anxious feeling like our wise country mouse: flee to the seaside, or countryside, or local park when you can. Eat sensibly, exercise, meditate, keep a journal, and seek out positive people and interactions to assist in your quest for relief from anxiety. And add CBD to this balanced and holistic template and live the anxiety-free life you thoroughly deserve.

DOSING CBD FOR STRESS & ANXIETY

People with constant anxiety might achieve better success with a long-acting oral regimen compared with routes with faster

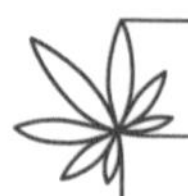

onset and shorter durations. However, those who suffer anxiety associated with acute pain attacks might find that inhalation can help achieve relief within minutes and prevent further anxiety. But you may consider multiple routes of administration for more complete symptom management.

A study published in 2019 suggested that a 25mg capsule of CBD, taken daily, significantly reduced anxiety in 47 of patients presenting with the primary concern of anxiety. If using THC, low doses (1–5mg) can be effective at reducing anxiety. It is important to be aware that if you are taking THC, doses of 10mg or more of THC can exacerbate anxiety.

It is important you seek medical advice if using CBD or cannabis to treat anxiety, especially if you are on prescription medication.

Finally, one in three of us live with some degree of anxiety every day. Let's lean into our bodies' natural abilities and defences to support our mental health but let's also remember…

Life is messy and we face challenges but whatever you do today let it be enough because we are all enough.

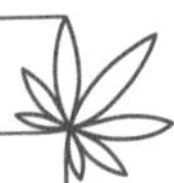

Exploring Sleep & CBD

More and more of us suffer from sleep disturbances! These can be associated with many factors including anxiety, chronic pain, depression, hormonal imbalances, stress, age, gender or substance abuse to name a few. The risks associated with persistent insomnia include increased risk of cardiovascular events, decreased immunity, diabetes, obesity, asthma, and seizures.

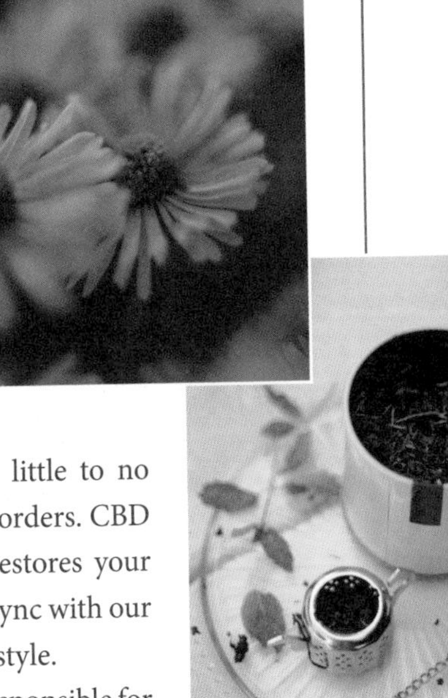

Many of us are turning to CBD as an effective treatment, with little to no side effects, for a range of sleeping disorders. CBD is a successful sleep aid because it restores your natural sleep cycle, which falls out of sync with our schedules in today's modern busy lifestyle.

Our endocannabinoid system is responsible for regulating our sleep as well as having many other

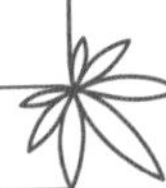

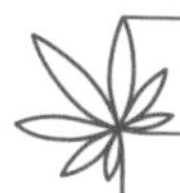

functions which all feed into the health of our sleep. Building a better relationship with sleep starts by seeking equilibrium within our endocannabinoid system.

WHAT HAPPENS IN THE BRAIN DURING SLEEP?

We know that brain chemicals are very involved in our sleep cycle. Neurotransmitters are chemicals that help the nerves communicate. They control whether we're awake or asleep, depending on which neurons they are acting upon. Neurons in the brainstem produce neurotransmitters, called serotonin and

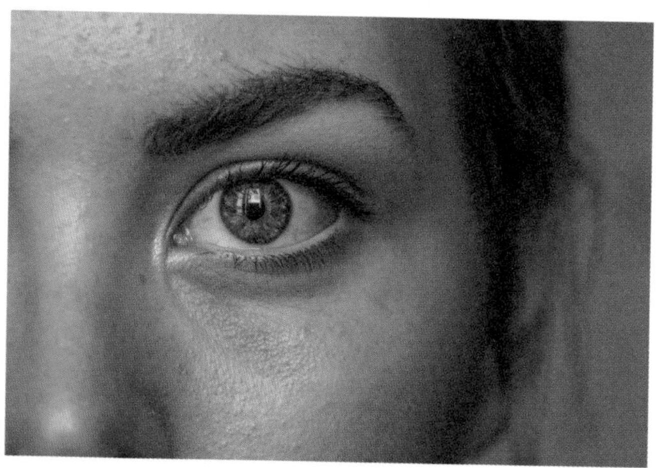

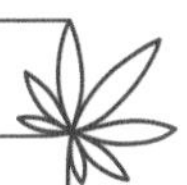

norepinephrine. These chemicals keep our brain active when we're awake, whereas neurons located at the base of the brain are responsible for us falling asleep. It seems these neurons turn off the signals that keep us awake.

An optimized endocannabinoid system, fuelled by CBD, helps to regulate these neurons and encourage unbroken sleep. Furthermore, if you don't get enough good quality sleep your health will suffer. Melatonin from your pineal gland is responsible for your circadian rhythm, in other words, when you sleep and wake, and for managing your energy levels. For most people, it's highest at night and lowest in the morning. A healthy endocannabinoid system is fundamental to the quality and wellbeing of your sleep pattern.

THE MECHANISMS OF SLEEP

In order to understand the benefits and potential power of CBD when tackling sleep issues, we first need to understand the complexities of sleep itself. We know that brain chemicals are very involved in our sleep cycle. Neurotransmitters are chemicals that help the nerves communicate. They control whether we're awake or asleep, depending on which neurons — our nerve cells — they're acting upon. There are neurons in the brainstem, where the brain and spinal cord meet, producing neurotransmitters

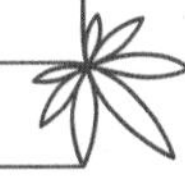

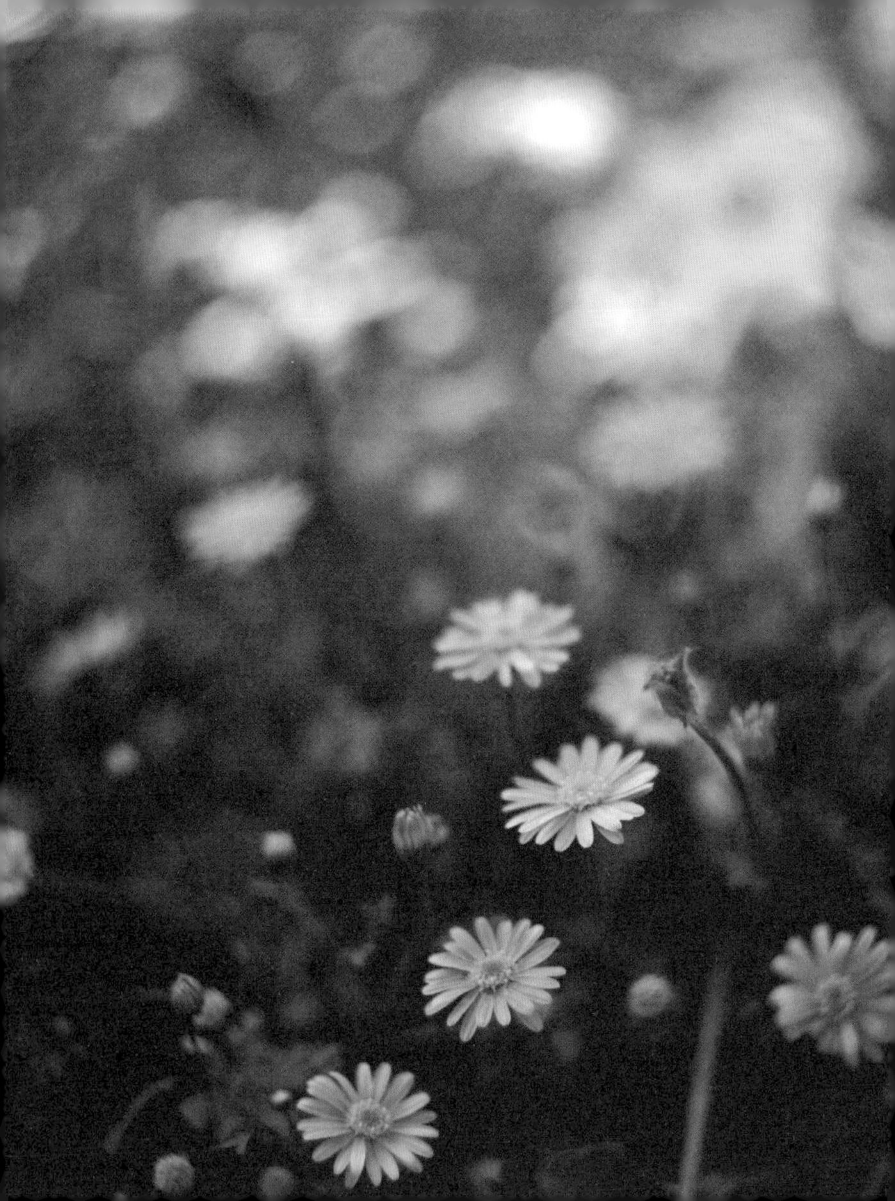

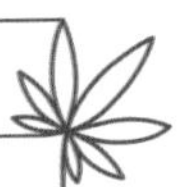

called serotonin and norepinephrine. These chemicals keep our brain active when we're awake. The neurons located at the base of the brain are responsible for us falling asleep. It seems these neurons turn off the signals that keep us awake.

When you sleep, your brain goes through natural cycles of activity. In healthy sleep, our rest is divided into four repeating stages: three of NREM (non-rapid eye movement) and one of REM (rapid eye movement) sleep.

NREM sleep happens first and includes three stages, the third stage of which is our deepest and is crucial to the efficient recuperation of our entire being. The last stage of NREM sleep is when you sleep most deeply. It's hard to wake up from this stage. This is followed by the intense dream state of the REM phase, during which our bodies are temporarily paralyzed, and brain activity markedly increases. REM sleep happens later in the night through to wakefulness, and can be vivid enough to make crossing the threshold into the start of the day as confusing as it is often unwelcome – it's as if the early morning dream state is preparing us for the busy day ahead with some gymnastic mental rehearsals.

As you sleep, your body cycles through these stages of NREM and REM sleep. You start the sleep cycle with stage 1 of NREM sleep, you pass through the other stages of NREM sleep

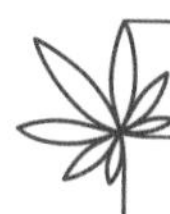

followed by a short period of REM sleep, then the cycle begins again at stage 1. A full sleep cycle takes about 90 to 110 minutes. Your first REM period is short. As the night goes on, you'll have longer REM sleep and less deep sleep.

Let's take a deeper look at the three stages that make up NREM sleep. The first stage is light sleeping that lasts for five to ten minutes. Everything starts to slow down, including your eye movement and muscle activity. Your eyes stay closed. If you get woken from stage 1 sleep, you may feel as if you haven't slept at all. You may remember fragments of images. Sometimes, you may feel like you're starting to fall and then experience a sudden muscle contraction. Healthcare providers call this motion hypnic myoclonic or hypnic jerk. Hypnic jerks are common and not anything to be concerned about as this occurrence is unlikely to cause any complications or side effects.

Stage 2 is the period of light sleep that features periods of muscle tone (muscles partially contracting) mixed with periods of muscle relaxation. Your eye movement stops, heart rate slows and body temperature decreases. Brain waves become slower. Occasionally, you'll have a burst of rapid waves called sleep spindles and your body prepares to enter deep sleep.

Stage 3 is deep sleep. During this stage, your brain produces delta waves — very slow brain waves. It's hard for someone

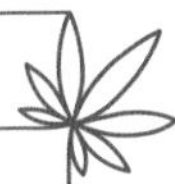

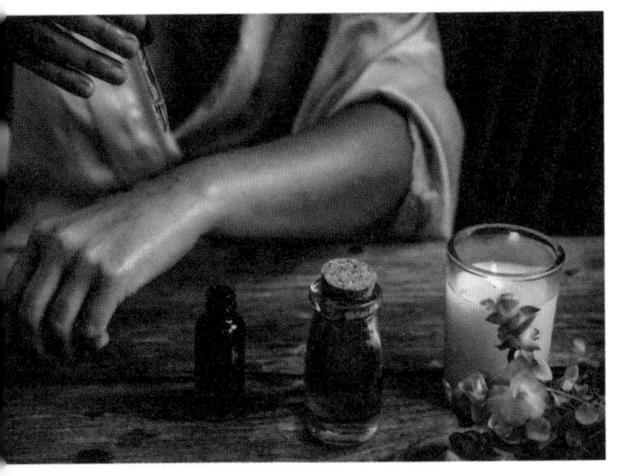

to wake you up during this stage, and you have no eye movement or muscle activity. If you're woken up, you may feel groggy and disoriented for a few minutes. During NREM stages, your body builds bone and muscle, repairs and regenerates tissues and strengthens the immune system. As you age, you get less NREM sleep. Older adults get less deep sleep than younger people.

On the other hand, when you enter REM sleep, brain activity increases again, meaning sleep is not as deep. The activity levels are like when you're awake. That's why REM sleep is the stage where you'll have intense dreams. At the same time, major muscles that you normally control (such as arms and legs) can't move. Usually, REM sleep arrives about an hour and a half after you go to sleep. The first REM period lasts about ten minutes. Each REM stage that follows gets longer and longer.

The amount of REM sleep you experience changes as you

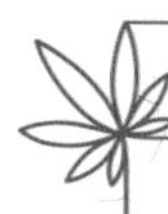

age. The percentage of REM sleep is highest during infancy and early childhood, it declines during adolescence and young adulthood and declines even more as you get older. Within your body during REM sleep, there is increased brain activity and muscle relaxation, your body goes through a series of changes, including faster breathing, increased heart rate and blood pressure, penile erections and rapid eye movement.

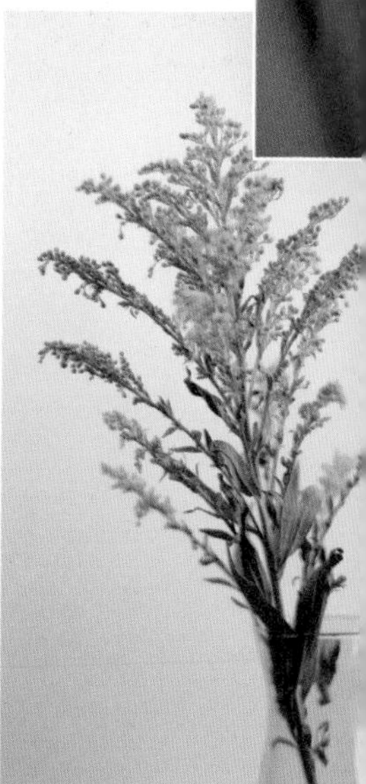

It is important to consider that chemical signals in the brain influence our sleep and wake cycles. Anything that shifts the balance of these neurotransmitters can make us feel drowsier or more awake. For example, alcohol may help people fall into a light sleep. But it reduces the deeper stages of sleep and REM sleep and leads to more disrupted sleep. Caffeine and pseudoephedrine can stimulate the brain. They may cause insomnia, an inability to sleep. Watch out for caffeinated drinks such as coffee and drugs such as diet pills and decongestants. Medications such as antidepressants can cause less REM sleep. People who smoke heavily often sleep lightly and have less REM sleep. They may wake up

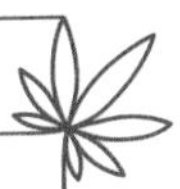

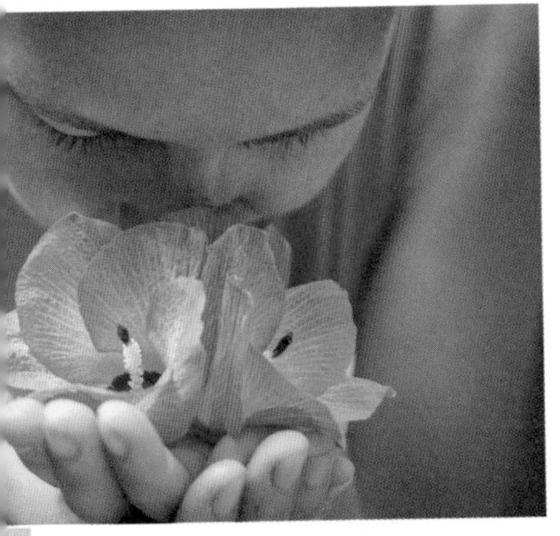

after a few hours because they experience nicotine withdrawal. Very hot or cold temperatures can also disrupt REM sleep. We're less able to regulate body temperature during REM sleep.

SLEEP HORMONES

If you don't get enough sleep, your health will suffer. Melatonin from your pineal gland is responsible for your circadian rhythm, in other words, when you sleep and wake, and for managing your energy levels. For most people, it's highest at night and lowest in the morning. A CBD-fuelled endocannabinoid system can affect sleep stability, how quickly you fall asleep and increases the level of melatonin produced.

LEANING INTO CBD TO AID SLEEP

Because of its effectiveness in treating both physical and emotional distress, CBD relaxes you and helps you more easily drift into normal, healthy sleep. The cannabinoids also trigger

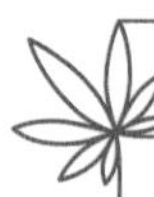

the release of the "sleep chemical" adenosine, which suppresses the brain's arousal system and promotes that luxurious feeling of sleepiness we all crave when desiring rest. However, there is evidence to suggest that at higher doses, CBD may have contrary effects, with CBD triggering an even deeper sleepiness. THC is believed to reduce the duration of REM sleep cycles, within which we experience our most intense dreams, and also process the mental data flow of our daily lives. This would appear to benefit to sufferers of PTSD (post-traumatic stress disorder), for whom dreams often become nightmares. But because our REM cycles are also important in regulating our immune systems, and maintaining healthy cognition, a balance must be struck between appropriate dosage and desired benefits.

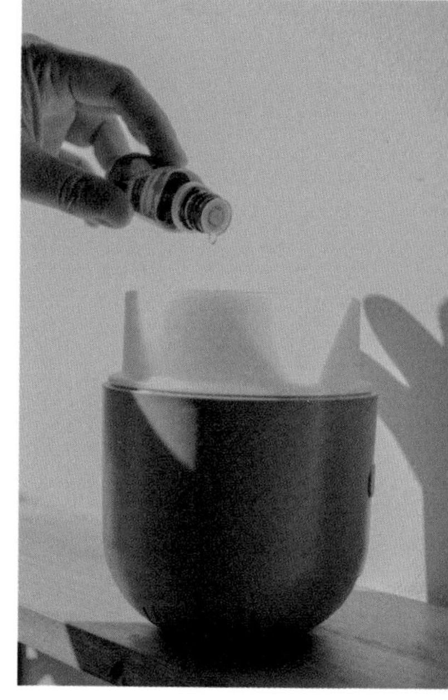

The same is true for CBD, which produces in some people a

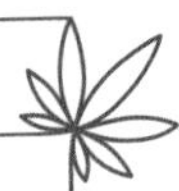

stimulant effect at low doses (which may make it suitable for the treatment of conditions such as Excessive Daytime Sleepiness Disorder). The key is to start with moderate doses, and journal your feelings daily about the different ways in which your mind and body respond. As little as 25mg of CBD oil a day, taken orally as a tincture or chewed as a gummy can have a noticeable effect on the quality of our sleep.

Before considering a CBD regimen, look at your sleep hygiene, including pre-sleep habits, sleep-wake cycle, all sleep-related complaints, and the impact of these events during the day. Timing is important when it comes to using CBD, especially for sleep. For some it can take about one hour to kick in and for others it can be closer to two to three hours. It can also affect us for longer than intended and cause grogginess in the morning. In my experience, one hour before bedtime is an ideal time to take your CBD. It will work for about three to four hours, helping you to fall asleep. It is vitally important you seek medical advice if using cannabis to treat sleep disturbances, especially if you are on prescription medication.

When used thoughtfully, and with patience, CBD may "knit up the ravelled sleeves" of our worry, and thus protect us from the murderous disruption of restlessness and insomnia.

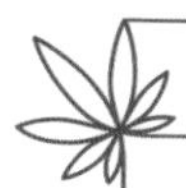

WHY THE QUALITY OF YOUR SLEEP MATTERS?

'...The innocent sleep,
Sleep that knits up the ravelled sleeve of care,
The death of each day's life, sore labour's bath,
Balm of hurt minds, great nature's second course,
Chief nourisher in life's feast.'

This extraordinary passage from Shakespeare's *Macbeth*, spoken in regret by the play's murderous protagonist after he has committed the first of his horrifying crimes — he fears he has murdered sleep itself, as well as his victims — is literature's most beautiful evocation of the sacred importance of sleep in our lives. Sleep rebuilds our minds, soothes our pain, nourishes our souls. Without it, we are incomplete.

According to the UK's National Health Service, "Regular poor sleep puts you at risk of serious medical conditions, including obesity, coronary heart disease and diabetes - and it shortens your life expectancy." A RAND Europe study estimates the cost to US productivity as a result of lost sleep to be over $400 billion, and in excess of a million American workdays. Sleep deprivation hits our bodies and our wallets equally hard. Sleep should come easily — when we're tired, we're tired — but

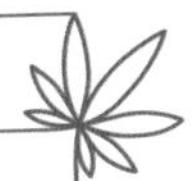

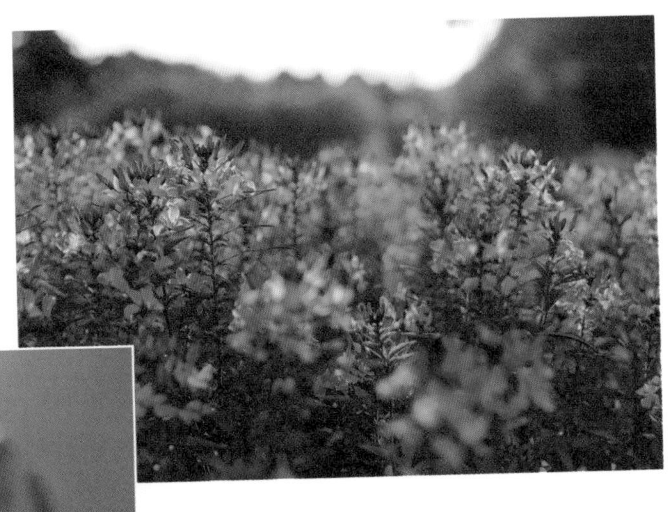

the reality of our busy lives is that circumstances often seem to conspire to make it close to impossible. In addition to illness, sleep disorders and medications, stress and anxiety can regularly threaten this 'balm of hurt minds', and deny us the relief from the discomfort these conditions have themselves brought about.

Pain, Inflammation & CBD

CBD has powerful anti-inflammatory therapeutic properties for our skin and body, and it can help with pain relief in four main ways. It tackles inflammation, which contributes to pain; it reduces anxiety, which is often experienced alongside

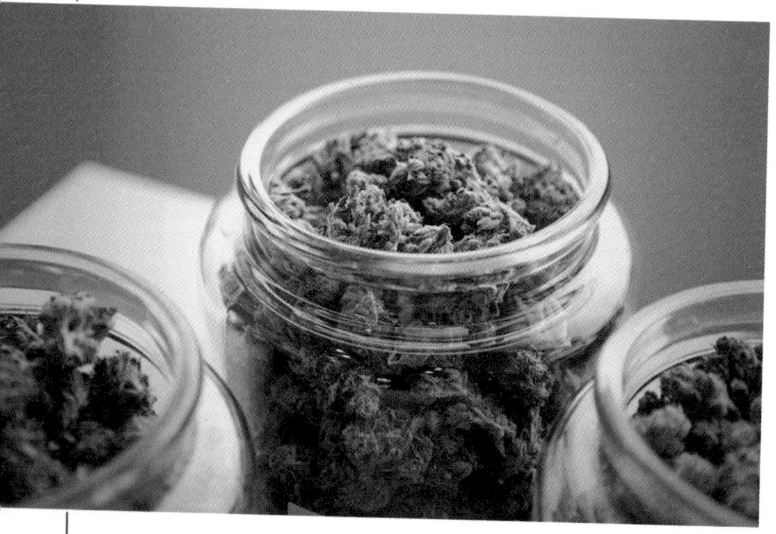

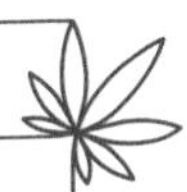

chronic pain; and it interrupt's the "I'm in pain" messages our body sends to our brain, diminishing our perception of the pain. Also, CBD can provide analgesia by impacting the manner in which nerves communicate pain signals. Pretty smart plant ingredient, right?

Chronic pain is one of the main reasons why people reach for medical cannabis and CBD. The compound's analgesic effect has some of the most robust research underpinning it, both pharmacologically and clinically. Activation of the endocannabinoid system by feeding it CBD, both centrally and peripherally, has been found to reduce both the perception of pain and the inflammation triggering the pain signal. Combined with the effects of cannabinoids on the many other previously mentioned receptor systems involved in pain signalling and perception, this means that the cannabinoids constitute a variety of redundant pathways, all contributing towards the end result of pain relief.

There are a number of receptors and processes involved in the experience of pain, many of which are influenced by CBD. As an analgesic, CBD is able to target the perception of pain through its activation of endocannabinoid receptors, which also reduces nociception – the detection of painful stimuli. It is not just the perception of pain that is influenced, but also the cause of pain. The tissue damage and swelling involved in

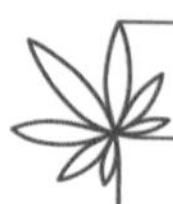

inflammation causes pain through the release of cytokines, as well as various hormone-like compounds utilized by our body to send pain signals.

Neuropathic pain is often caused by damage to the nervous system, whether through trauma, stress, chemotherapy, or infection. One thing that can happen here is an increase in the release of neurotransmitters such as glutamate, which can cause sensations of pain and nerve damage. This can also trigger surrounding nerve cells to increase their firing as well. CBD has been shown to be an effective intervention here as well, as it stimulates the firing of faster A-beta nerve fibres, which increase endorphins and reduce the perception of chronic pain. There is also the category of dysfunctional pain, in which no damage to the nervous system or inflammation is apparent, yet there is still intense pain. CBD has been found to alleviate symptoms of these conditions in many cases.

Other areas where CBD is being effectively used to treat pain is in cancer treatment relief, especially when treating the side effects of chemotherapy. It is also a popular solution for arthritic pain and migraines. The dose of CBD for each case is unique to the patients taking CBD but 5–10mg of CBD daily seems to be a successful starting point.

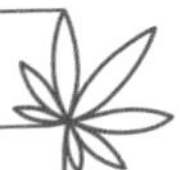

CBD, Sex and Confidence

CBD and sex are best friends! CBD increases blood flow to tissues, which increases nerve sensitivity, helping to make sex more pleasurable while intensifying your orgasm. It also promotes the body's own natural lubrication. CBD will help reduce anxiety, helping you get out of your head and back in touch with your beautiful sexy self. But when we understand our own ability to be sexually confident, we really start to win in our own skin.

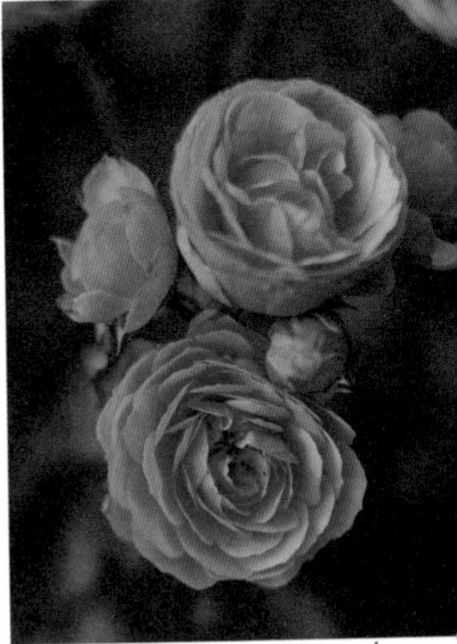

Sexual confidence is not about how good you are in bed, it's more about how comfortable you feel in your body. But feeling comfortable in your body does not always come naturally: it's not always that easy to achieve and definitely not all the time. But one thing is for sure: feeling confident and comfortable in your own skin starts with self-love, self-appreciation, and self-acceptance.

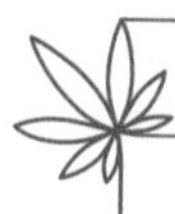

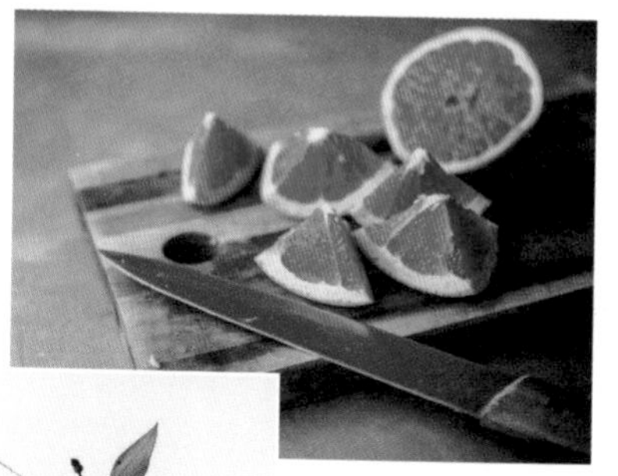

The level of philosophy, theory and intellectual conversation around sexual confidence, sexual wellbeing and sexual growth has exponentially increased and became much less of a taboo (thankfully) in the last few years. And this can only be great news, especially for women, whose bodies are designed to evolve, to create miracles, and to serve us in ways that are profoundly challenging but also astonishingly beautiful. I'm not going to jump completely into the psychology of sexual confidence but there is one nugget of knowledge that I find super interesting. This might give you some insight into your own sexual confidence, no matter your gender, age or sexual preferences.

There is a concept within sexual education relating to our sex drive (or lack

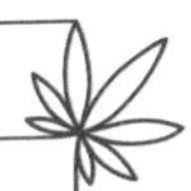

of) which is fascinating! This concept relates to two things, our sexual accelerators (turn ons) or sexual brakes (turn offs). If you naturally have a heavy foot on your sexual accelerator, you tend to crave sex and enjoy sex more, you will find small details about your partner exciting and you will have a greater interest in sex generally. Sexual brakes on the other hand can be influenced by internal or external factors. Your sexual brakes can be triggered by stress, the need for protection, trauma, an unsafe and/or uncomfortable environment, or maybe you're just not feeling it.

We all have a sexual accelerator and a sexual brake; both are important to have and we have different levels of both. This can change throughout our life, depending on so many factors.

Regardless of how in tune you feel with your accelerator or brake, self-confidence is key. It can fuel the accelerator and reinforce self-respect, which keeps the brakes at hand in case we need to create safe boundaries. And remember: boundaries are sexy!

The great news is CBD is wonderful as a sexual ally, but equally so in building self-confidence as it reduces our stress and creates space in our mind for our own self-love practice.

Remember, CBD is a powerful anti-inflammatory and can increase blood flow while helping to relax muscles. These properties make CBD a great natural lubricant for sex.

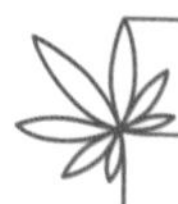

Furthermore, some women even say they experience heightened sensation and better orgasms by using CBD as their lubricant.

CBD AND YOUR LIBIDO

CBD could help you in the bedroom and have a positive effect on your libido. There are lots of reports and research supporting the theory that CBD can boost libido and increase lubrication during sex. We already know that CBD is a stress buster and dramatically reduces anxiety, which will help your mindset from a sexual point of view. Before you rush out to stock up on CBD products for the nightstand, lets strip this right back and look at what the scientific evidence really says and discover how researchers think CBD affects our bodies.

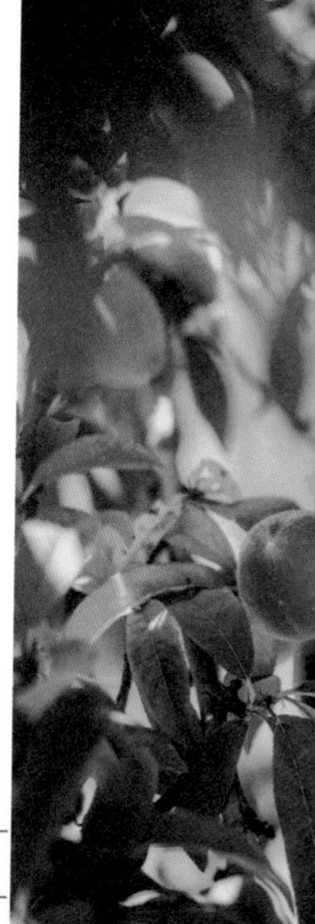

The ECS, although only discovered in the early 1990s, is a complex cell-signalling system connected throughout our body as well as to the reproductive organs and sexual tissue. Our bodies produce cannabinoids naturally, these cannabinoids are called endocannabinoids. We also produce two receptors called CB1 and CB2,

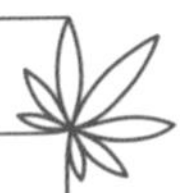

which are located in the ECS. CB2 receptors are often found in our immune cells and primarily impact pain and inflammation, whereas CB1 receptors are more commonly found in the brain.

A study published in December 2013 showed results of a significant relationship between endocannabinoid concentrations and female sexual arousal. There is little scientific research available on CBD lubricants, which means that most of what we know about CBD lubricants and sexual pleasure is anecdotal. This is what we do know though: one of the major hero ingredients in many skincare lines today is CBD, due to its anti-inflammatory and therapeutic properties when applied topically. When ingested, it has the same anti-inflammatory properties.

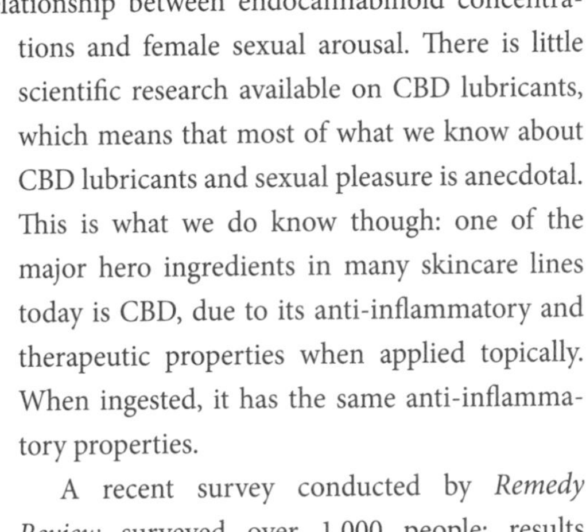

A recent survey conducted by *Remedy Review* surveyed over 1,000 people: results showed that 68% of people said CBD improved their sexual experience. Adding a CBD-infused lubricant could: make sex more comfortable and improve sexual performance, relieving pain for those who struggle with dryness and painful sex by increasing blood flow to tissues; increase

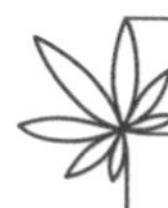

sensitivity, and promote the body's own natural lubrications. Anxiety about your sexual performance is normal and common in us all at different times in our sexual journey. When our sexual anxiety is visiting, our libido leaves the building, simply adding to more stress and anxiety between the sheets. The desire for sex may go up when this anxiety is calmed. Some scientists believe that CBD can affect sexual desire directly in the brain. A recent open-randomized study of 21 heterosexuals, assessed the aphrodisiacal properties of cannabis. The authors concluded that using cannabis may be helpful for people with a low sex drive.

WHAT ABOUT OUR HORMONES?

Our hormones are incredibly powerful forces within our biology. They will affect and impact our mood, appetite, fertility, sex drive, metabolism and energy levels. They form a communication network that gives and receives constant feedback, which helps maintain our optimal bodily function and homeostasis. Hormonal imbalance happens when the communication network breaks down. CBD feeds our endocannabinoid system whose job is literally to restore and maintain homeostasis.

Our hormones are responsible for essentially every function in our bodies. Hormones are chemicals secreted by our glands

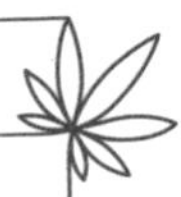

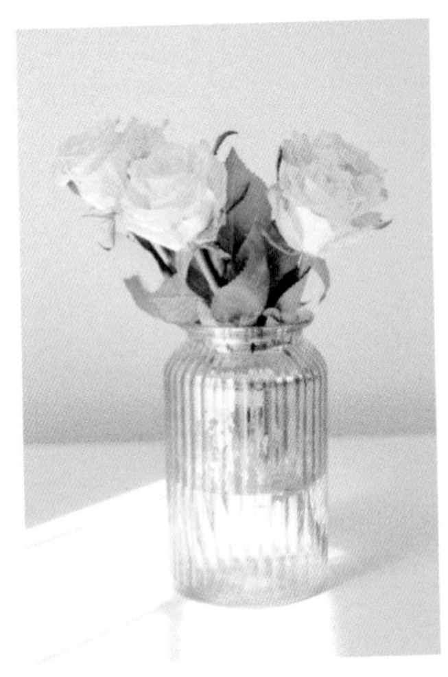

in order to send "messages" through the bloodstream. Those messages then tell our organs what to do to keep us alive and healthy. When we think "hormone", we usually think about the sex hormones, testosterone or oestrogen, but there are actually more than 50 different hormones circulating inside your body right now.

When your hormones are balanced and working in sync, you won't notice them, of course, and that's a good thing. It's when they're imbalanced that you could start seeing cascading health issues take over. Hormonal imbalance stems from your body making too little or too much of a hormone or a series of hormones. There are many hormones, such as insulin or adrenaline, that everyone shares, but specific hormones can affect men and women in different ways. For example, women may see an imbalance in oestrogen and progesterone levels, while men may experience an imbalance in testosterone.

You have experienced – or are likely to – a hormonal imbalance at some point in your life, especially if you have an endocrine disorder. Age and lifestyle are factors, too. The symptoms of hormonal imbalance can vary widely, as each hormone is uniquely responsible for its role.

THE CORE HORMONES

Oestrogen is one of the main sex hormones in women. While men have oestrogen too, they secrete smaller amounts and do not experience the same effects from oestrogen that women do. In women, oestrogen is responsible for the physical changes during puberty, regulating your menstrual cycle and supporting your bones, heart and mood during pregnancy. In both men and women, oestrogen helps to regulate cholesterol and bone health.

The progesterone hormone is generally assumed to be only present in women, but men have progesterone as well. For women, progesterone is crucial in menstruation and supporting the early stages of pregnancy. For men, progesterone helps support fertility and balances the effects of oestrogen on the body.

Testosterone is the main sex hormone in men. While women also have testosterone, they have smaller amounts and do not experience the same effects from testosterone that men do. For

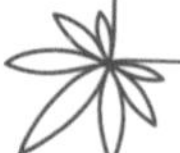

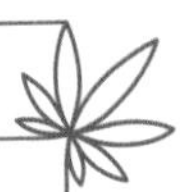

men, testosterone supports the physical changes during puberty, such as deepening of the voice and growth of the genitals, hair and muscles. In women, testosterone supports bone health and reproductive tissue.

The hormone insulin is produced by the pancreas and allows your muscles, fat and liver to absorb glucose, also referred to as blood sugar, and breakdown fat and protein in order to regulate your metabolic process. An imbalance can cause, not only diabetes, but heart

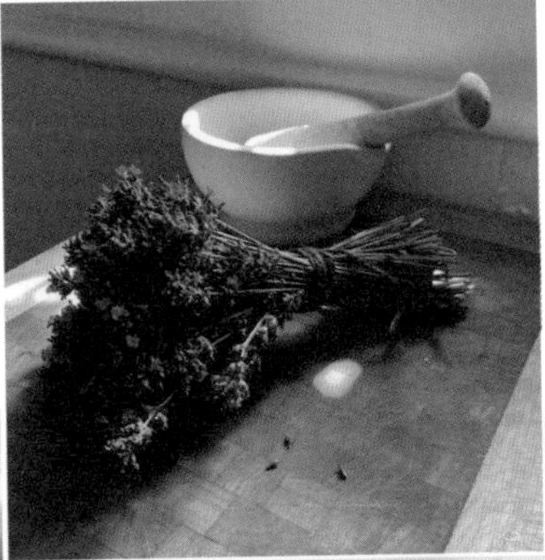

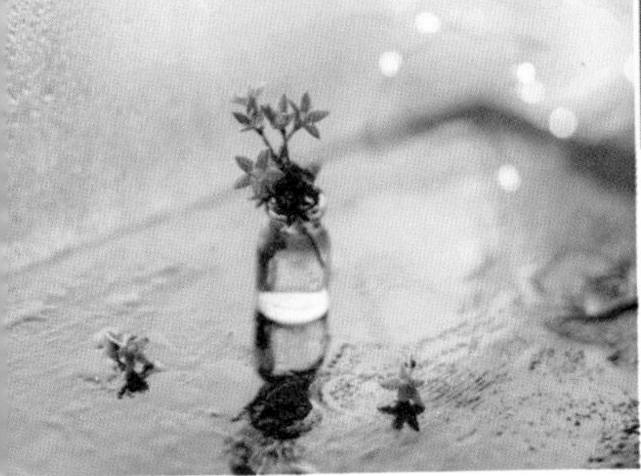

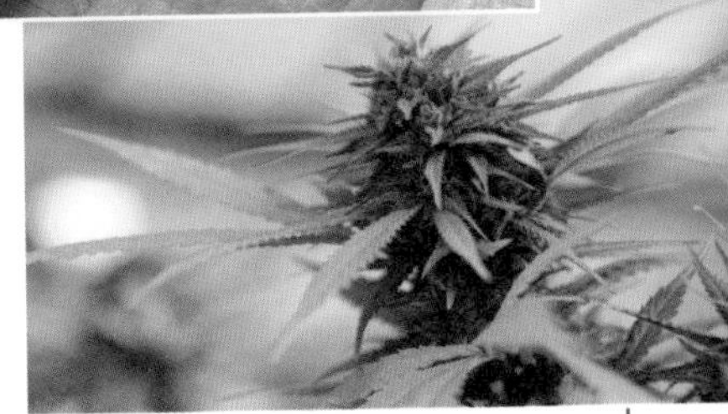

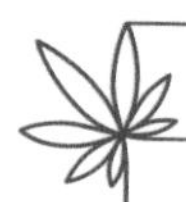

disease and obesity. We know that cannabinoid consumption seems to be related to reduced blood-sugar levels. Furthermore, research shows that when diabetic people use medicinal cannabis, they can reduce their diabetic medicine or insulin, as cannabinoids lower blood glucose.

The endocannabinoid system's primary function is to control how your body releases the neurotransmitters that affect nerve impulses. The ECS is known to regulate stress, mood, memory, fertility, bone growth, pain, immune function, among other things. CBD interacts with the ECS and with many other receptors in the body. CBD can influence major hormones, including insulin, cortisol, and melatonin. The way that CBD and the ECS work are complicated and further research is needed, but there is some evidence to suggest that CBD could help with the symptoms of a hormone imbalance.

Our mood, personality, outlook on life, energy levels and ability to cope is all hormonal. Once we begin to understand that and explore how our hormones impact so much of our life, the more control we gain over so much of our day-to-day experiences.

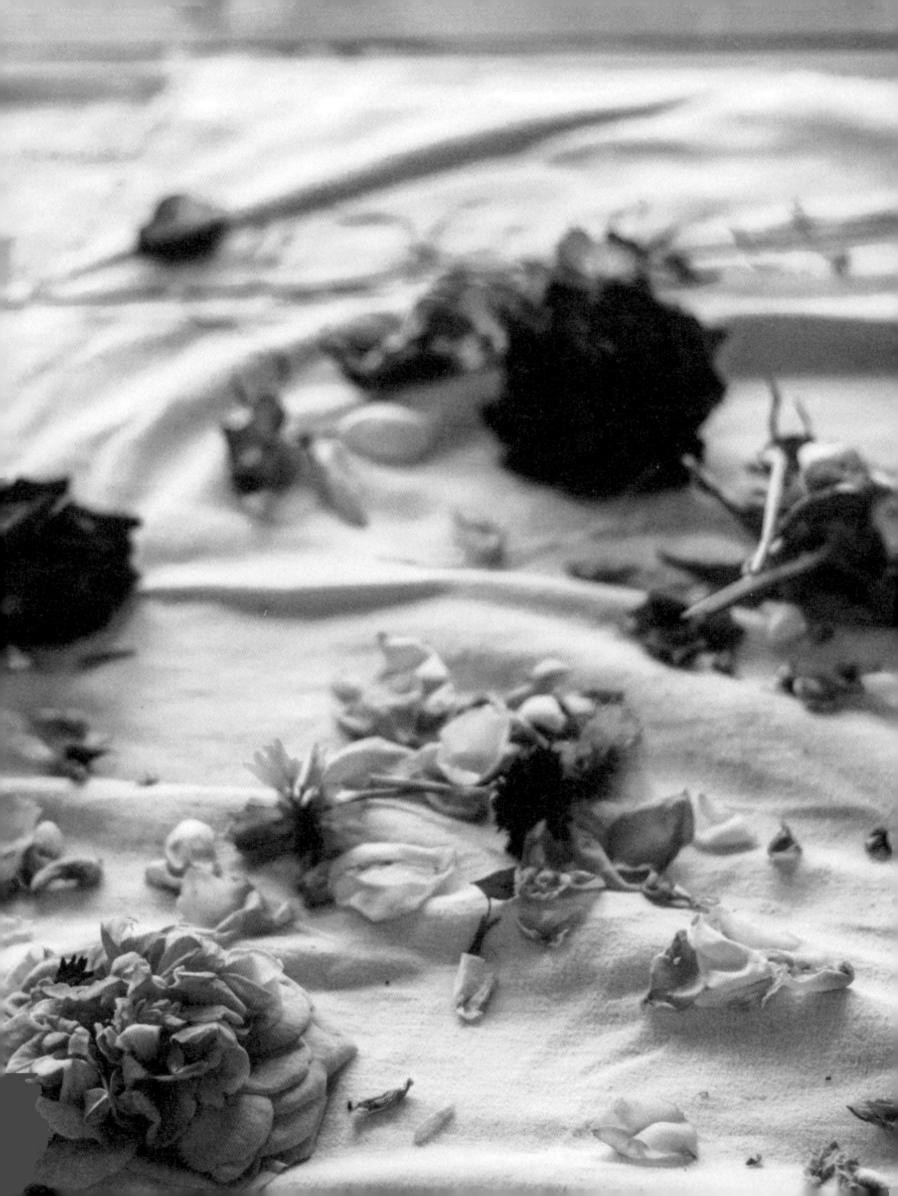

CHAPTER THREE

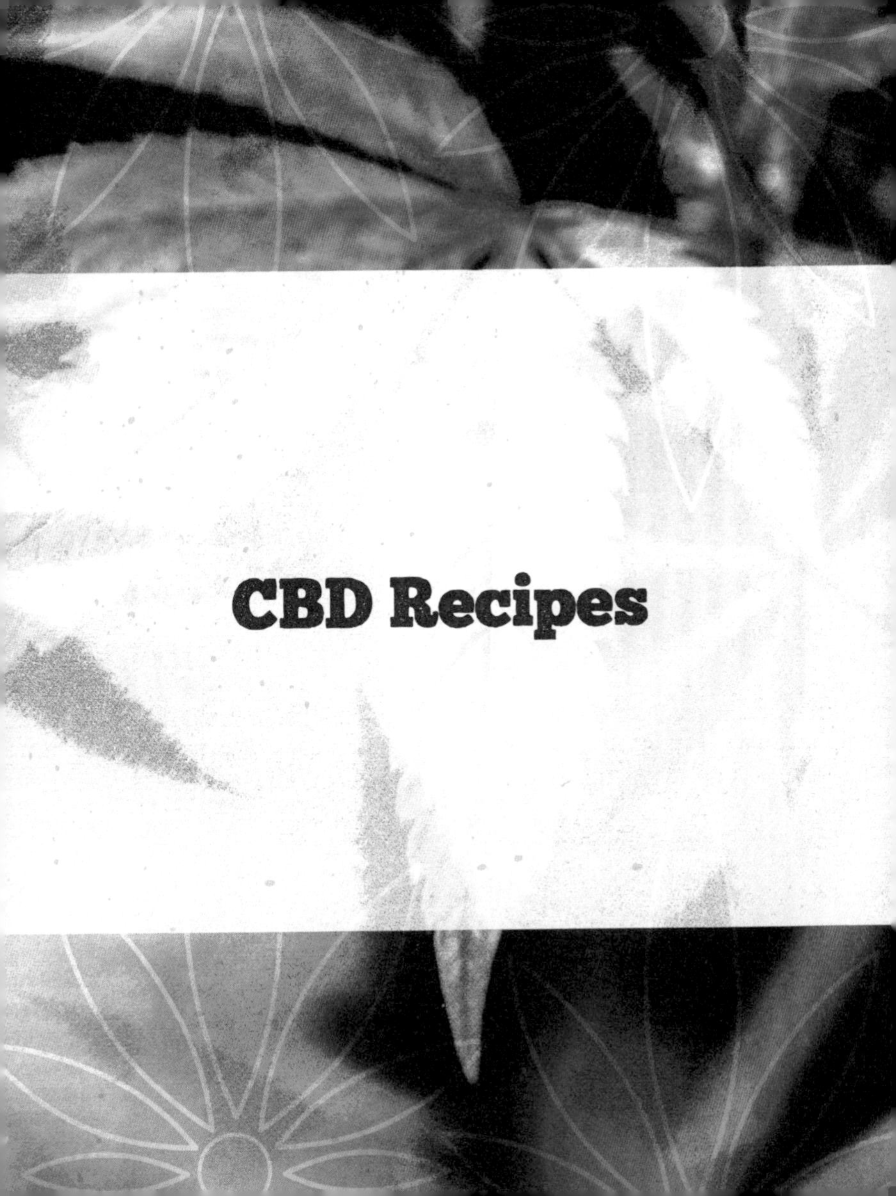

CBD Recipes

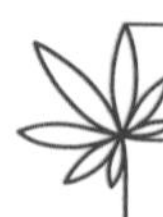

Making your own products using CBD is one of the most creative, fun and simple ways to tap into the therapeutic benefits of CBD, regardless of whether you're treating anxiety, pain, sleep disturbances or are leaning into the benefit of CBD for a happier, healthy sex life. As you step into your blending kitchen and get started, it is worth remembering that CBD is incredibly nourishing to your skin as well as having boundless health benefits. As we mentioned previously in this book, it offers powerful antioxidant and anti-inflammatory results that your skin will thank you for daily. These recipes cover an array of conditions and offer a variety of solutions. I've designed these recipes to be simple, easy to make and amazingly effective – so dive in and get creative by formulating your own.

Given that so many recipes in this book combine CBD and essential oils, it is interesting to note that celebrated neurologist, Dr Ethan Russo says "research implies that the combined use of essential oils and cannabinoids may be a potential novel therapy for the treatment of neurodegeneration, and associated symptoms."

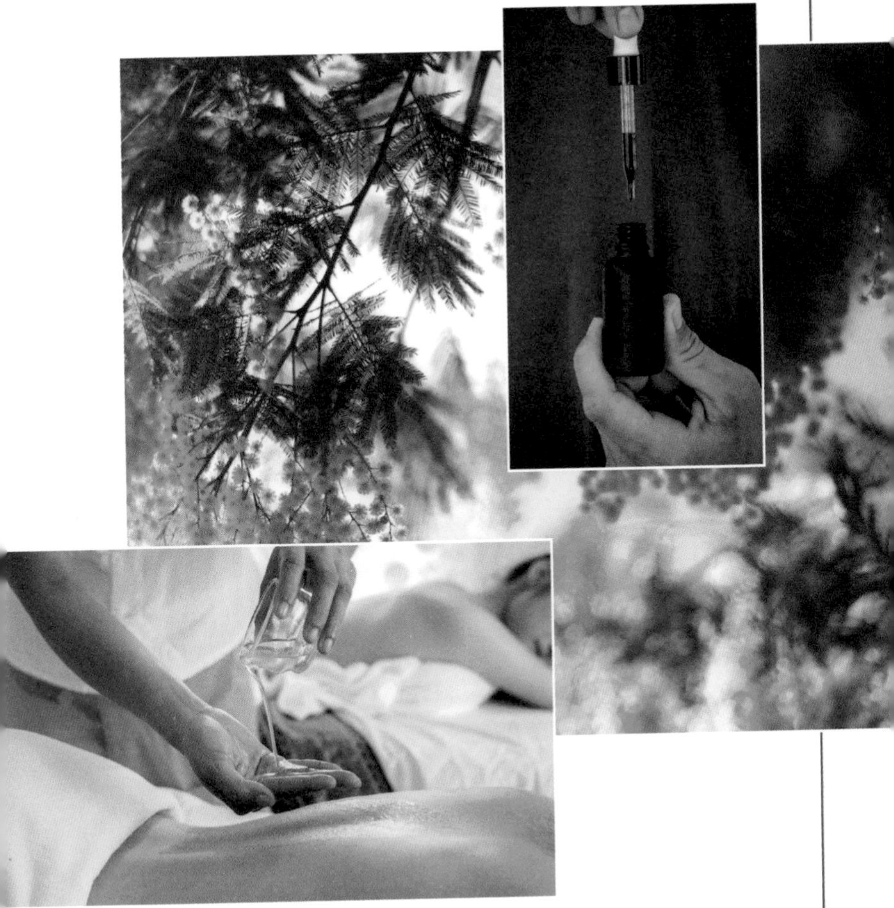

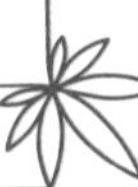

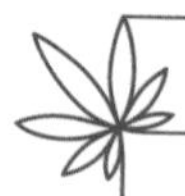

CBD Recipes

Before you run to the kitchen to start creating healthy wonderment with CBD, let's get you up to speed with a few key pieces of information to make your recipe-making process as smooth as possible.

Firstly, you won't need any special equipment for the recipes in this book. Most of what you need to make these recipes is already in your kitchen cupboard — for example, bowls, spoons and scales — however, I would highly recommend that you use a separate set of blending equipment for your CBD recipes as the essential oils can leave a lasting smell and taste on the equipment, and you don't want your food to taste of aromatherapy.

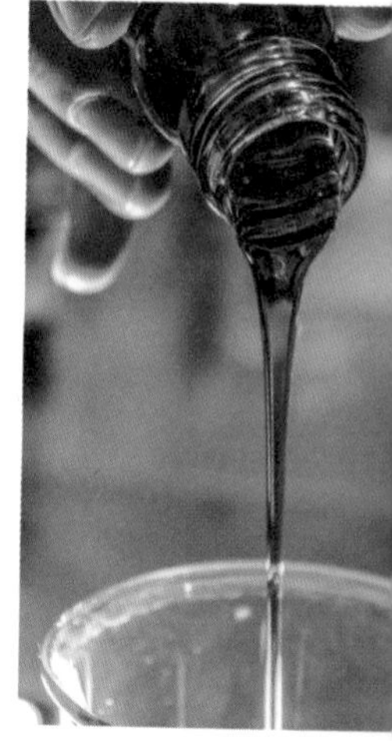

Here is what you will need for these CBD recipes:

Digital kitchen scale: because some of the ingredient amounts are small, a digital scale will be required to ensure the accuracy of your measurements.

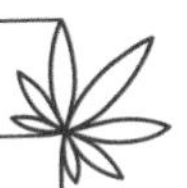

Measuring jugs: stainless steel and glass will be super helpful. I don't recommend plastic for multiple reasons but mostly the scent of the oil can last in plastic but will not in glass or stainless steel. Also both glass and stainless steel are quick to clean and easily sterilized.

Glass bowl and beaker: glass beakers will give you an easy pour for the oil-based recipes. They are easy to clean and sterilize.

Stirrer: you will need a stirrer or spoon for many of the recipes. I prefer glass or stainless steel again as it is easier to clean, but a wooden stirrer will also be fine.

Kitchen grater: you will need a standard grater to grate the cocoa butter for the bath soak recipe.

Double Boiler: when melting butters and waxes or gently heating vegetable oils you will need to use a double boiler. This can be achieved by simply heating a saucepan half filled with water, in which you place a stainless steel bowl or beaker containing the ingredient you are melting/heating into the water. The water in the sauce pan is the heat source needed to melt and heat the ingredients in the bowl.

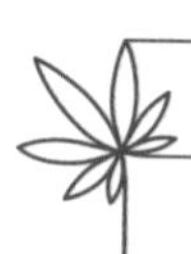

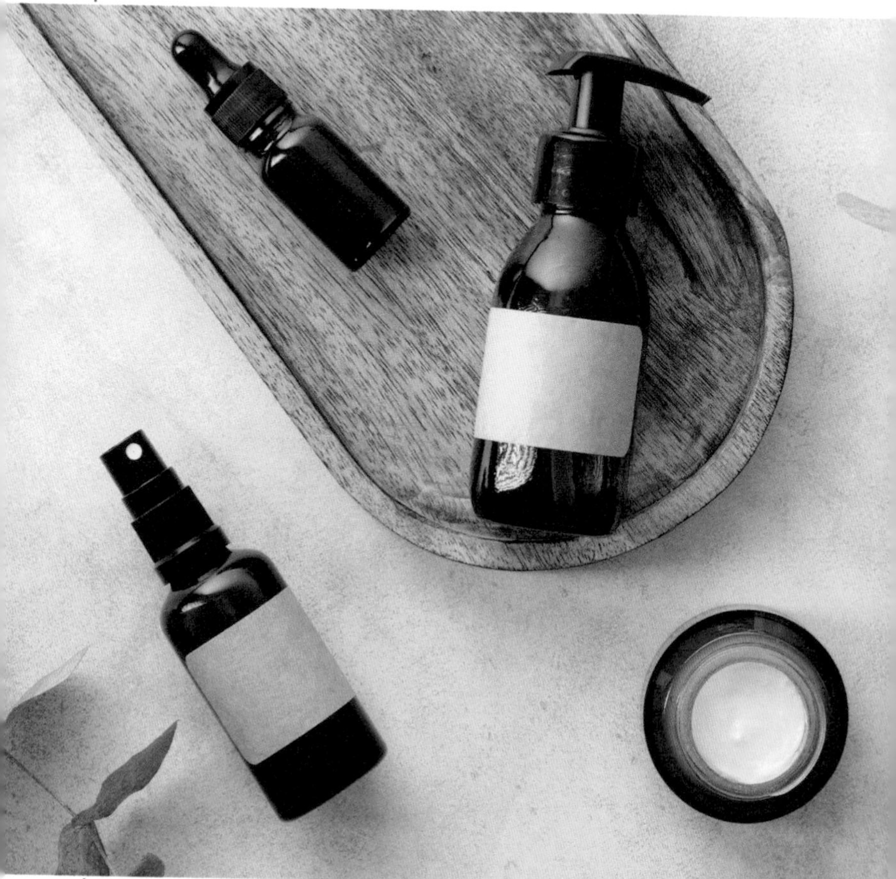

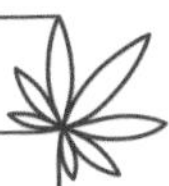

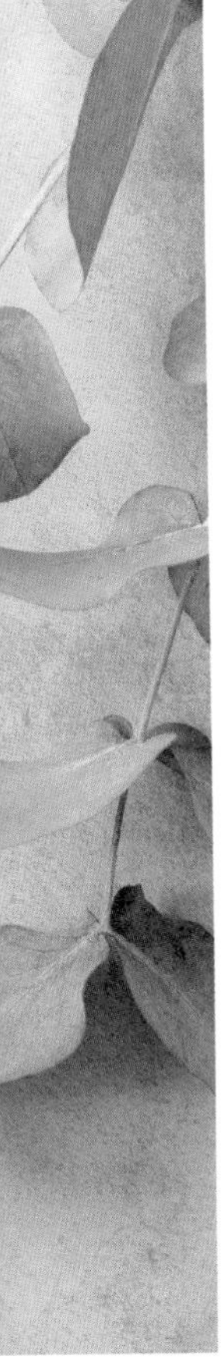

STORING YOUR INGREDIENTS AND RECIPES.

I keep my CBD oil, vegetable oil and essential oils in dark glass bottles or jars (either amber, navy or dark green), storing them in a cool, dry cupboard and making sure to seal them tightly after each use. For storing my completed recipes, I use glass containers as they will protect the natural ingredients from sunlight damage and keep your recipe fresh for longer. They are also beautiful as you can easily find different colours and shapes of glass containers online (suggested sites are listed below).

With each recipe, I offer advice on how long the product will stay fresh and how to store it. Oils, balms and salve products are typically not susceptible to mould caused by microbial and bacterial activity so they tend to have a two-to-six month shelf life, but be advised – over time they will oxidize and eventually turn rancid. They will all keep fresh for two months if you keep them cool and away from direct heat and sunlight. I always store oils in dark bottle to protect them from the day they are created. If you want to make bigger batches and extend your product's shelf life, add 1% of vitamin E to your recipe. Vitamin E is a natural antioxidant that will bring an additional layer of protection to your recipe.

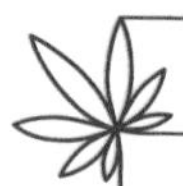

Supplier Suggestions

You wont need anything extraordinary to make these recipes but you may need to buy some essential oils, which you don't always have on hand. Below I share my most trusted suppliers: some I have loved for years, others are more recent favourites. I have listed global suppliers to help you find the best options, no matter where in the world you will be cooking up a CBD-inspired aromatically divine storm.

CBD SOURCES

cbii-cbd.com .... UK/EU
rosebudcbd.com .... US
shop-poplar.com .... US/UK/EU/CA/ROW
bloomfarmscbd.com .... US
charlottesweb.com .... US
blacktiecbd.net .... US
love-hemp.com .... UK/EU
cbd-guru.co.uk .... UK/EU/ROW
junepure.com .... EU/UK

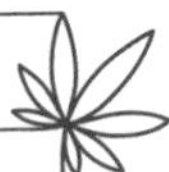

ESSENTIAL OILS

verdon-rosesetaromes.com . . . . EU/UK/US/CA/ROW
lessenteursduclaut.fr . . . . EU/UK/US/CA/ROW
essentianobilis.com . . . . EU/UK/US/CA/ROW
aromatics.com . . . . US/UK/EU/CA/ROW
oshadhi.co.uk . . . . UK/EU
newdirectionsaromatics.ca . . . . US/CA
escents.ca . . . . US/CA
edensgarden.com . . . . US/UK/EU/CA/ROW
baseformula.com . . . . UK

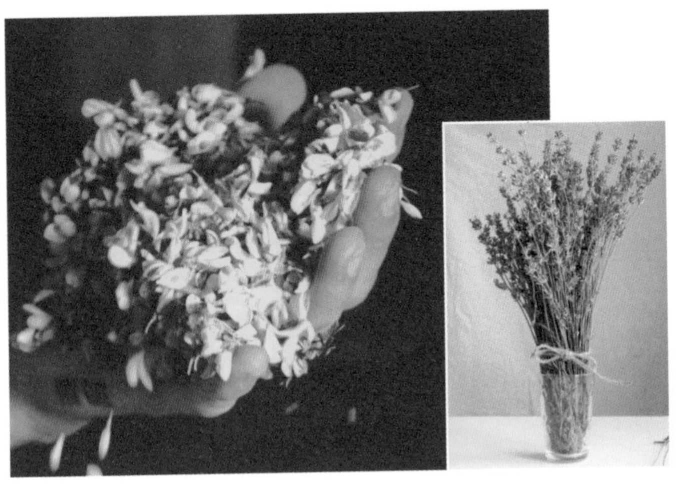

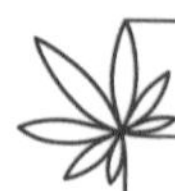

VEGETABLE OILS

aromatics.com .... US/UK/EU/CA/ROW
baldwins.co.uk .... UK/EU
nobleroots.com.. US
baseformula.com .... UK

BUTTERS AND WAXES

aromatics.com .... US/UK/EU/CA/ROW
hollandandbarrett.com .... UK/EU
thesoapkitchen.co.uk .... UK/EU
mountainroseherbs.com .... US/CA
organic-creations.com .... US
baseformula.com ....UK

HYDROSOLS

verdon-rosesetaromes.com .... EU/UK/US/CA/ROW
lessenteursduclaut.fr .... EU/UK/US/CA/ROW
essentianobilis.com .... EU/UK/US/CA/ROW
aromatics.com .... US/UK/EU/CA/ROW
edenbotanicals.com .... US/CA
mountainroseherbs.com .... US/CA

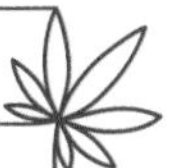

EQUIPMENT

walmart.com . . . . US
crateandbarrel.com . . . . US/UK
makingcosmetics.com . . . . US
zedmed.co.uk . . . . UK/EU
ikea.com . . . . UK/EU

CONTAINERS

ampulla.co.uk . . . . UK
lesamesfleurs.com . . . . CA
stocksmetic.com . . . . US/UK/CA
amazon.com . . . . UK/US/EU/CA/ROW

CBD AND ESSENTIAL OILS LEARNING RESOURCES

labaroma-education.com
labaroma-education.com/LabCBD
labaroma.com/podcast
projectcbd.org
essenceofthyme.com/programs

Stress Recipes

CBD DESTRESS ROLLER

Roller-ball recipes are one of the aromatherapy world's best kept secrets. A roller ball is a small, normally 10ml, bottle with a rolling ball insert and then a screw cap on top. The bottle is normally filled with a vegetable base oil and a selection of essential oils. One of the reasons this little product is so effective is because of its convenience and its powerful relationship with the olfactory system. Your olfactory system is your sense of smell. We know from recent science that one of the greatest ways to support our central nervous system is by using aromatics through inhalation and our sense of smell.

Our sense of smell was once considered the Cinderella of our senses as it was not given much respect. Through scientific appraisal, however, we know now that our olfactory system is tremendously influential and important, especially when communicating with the brain.

Ingredients

9ml jojoba oil
2 drops CBD oil
2 drops bergamot essential oil

2 drops frankincense essential oil
2 drops lavender essential oil
2 drops palo santo essential oil

Method

1. Add 9ml of jojoba vegetable oil and CBD oil to the roller blend bottle.

2. Add to the roller bottle the drops for all four essential oils.

3. Apply the roller ball and then the cap. Shake to blend the vegetable and essential oils.

Directions for use

Apply to your pulses and when required especially when you feel signs of overwhelm and stress starting.

Equipment & Storage

10ml roller ball bottle.

In a dark glass bottle your roller ball blend will keep fresh for two to six months.

Alchemy Note

This recipe works best when you apply it as soon as you feel overwhelmed. The secret to a roller ball blend working super effectively is to apply the roller to the pulses in your wrists and take three deep, mindful inhalation breaths. These three deep breaths serve to calm your central nervous system while also helping to transport the therapeutic compounds from the aromatic oils into your olfactory system so your brain can start to recognize that you are actively trying to calm down, breathe and relieve stress.

STRESS FREE CBD MASSAGE OIL

The concept behind treating stress with massage is twofold. Firstly, you reap the benefits from the destressing aromatic essential oils and the calming CBD oil, but your muscles truly begin to relax through the art of touch, which is delivered via massage. Even self-massage is a beautifully effective way to treat stress as you are taking the time to slow down and loosen tight and tired muscles while feeding your olfactory and the endocannabinoid system with curative plants.

Ingredients

20ml sunflower oil
15ml argan oil
14ml CBD oil
6 drops neroli essential oil
6 drops ylang ylang essential oil
5 drops mandarin essential oil
5 drops lavender essential oil
4 drops jasmine essential oil

Method

1. Combine the sunflower, argan and CBD oils. Gently stir in the drops from all five essential oils.

2. Transfer the mixture to the glass bottle and seal with the lid.

Directions for use

Shake the blend before use. Massage into the skin for a relaxing aromatic massage.

Equipment & Storage

50ml glass bottle and lid
Stirrer
As there is no water content in this massage oil, it will keep for up to six months if stored away from direct sunlight and heat.

Alchemy Note

If the aroma of florals is more appealing to you than the scent of citrus, I recommend you add two extra drops of jasmine to this blend and reduce the neroli to four drops. This small recipe adjustment will give you a much more exotic, floral scent, which may be a more destressing aroma for you.

DESTRESS TINCTURE

One of the most effective ways to feed your endocannabinoid system with CBD is by taking a daily CBD tincture. However, the market is saturated with CBD products, and it can be very confusing to find a good quality, affordable CBD tincture, so making your own is a wonderful option. The benefit of taking the CBD tincture daily is that it consistently and kindly feeds your endocannabinoid system, which helps with overwhelm, anxiety and stress as well as offering those additional anti-inflammatory and antioxidant benefits to your body and mind.

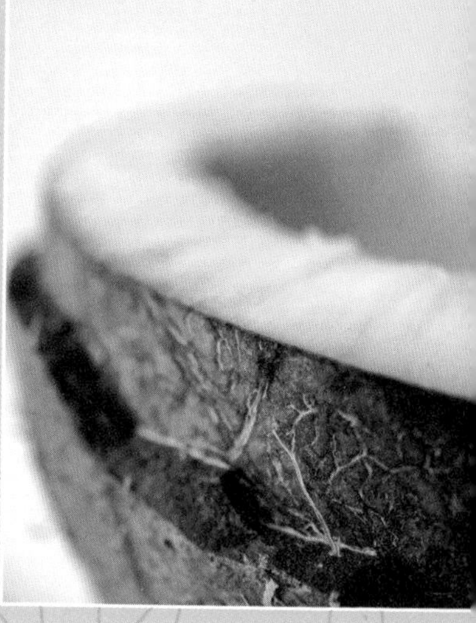

Ingredients

90grams coconut oil
10grams CBD isolate*

Method

1. Gently heat the coconut oil in a double boiler until 40°c.

2. Slowly stir in the CBD isolate until fully dissolved.

3. When cool, pour from stainless steel beaker into the 100ml glass bottle.

Directions for use

CBD is most effective when taken daily. I recommend you take five drops, up to three times a day. Take a moment and hold the drops under the tongue for 60 seconds before swallowing. Within this recipe with 10% CBD concentration, each drop is approximately 5mg CBD, the recommended 15 drops daily is 75mg.

Equipment & Storage

100ml glass ball bottle with pipette application
Stainless-steel beaker
Stirrer
Store in a cool location and away from natural light and your CBD tincture will last two to six months.

Alchemy Note

It can take a few weeks before you feel the benefits of taking CBD regularly, but everyone's body is different. Some people feel an impact in their day-to-day health within a week and for others it can take longer. Be patient and consistent with your new CBD routine.

**I have created this recipe using CBD isolate as growing your own hemp or cannabis in order to make a pure plant-based tincture may not be an available option for many due to legislation where you live.*

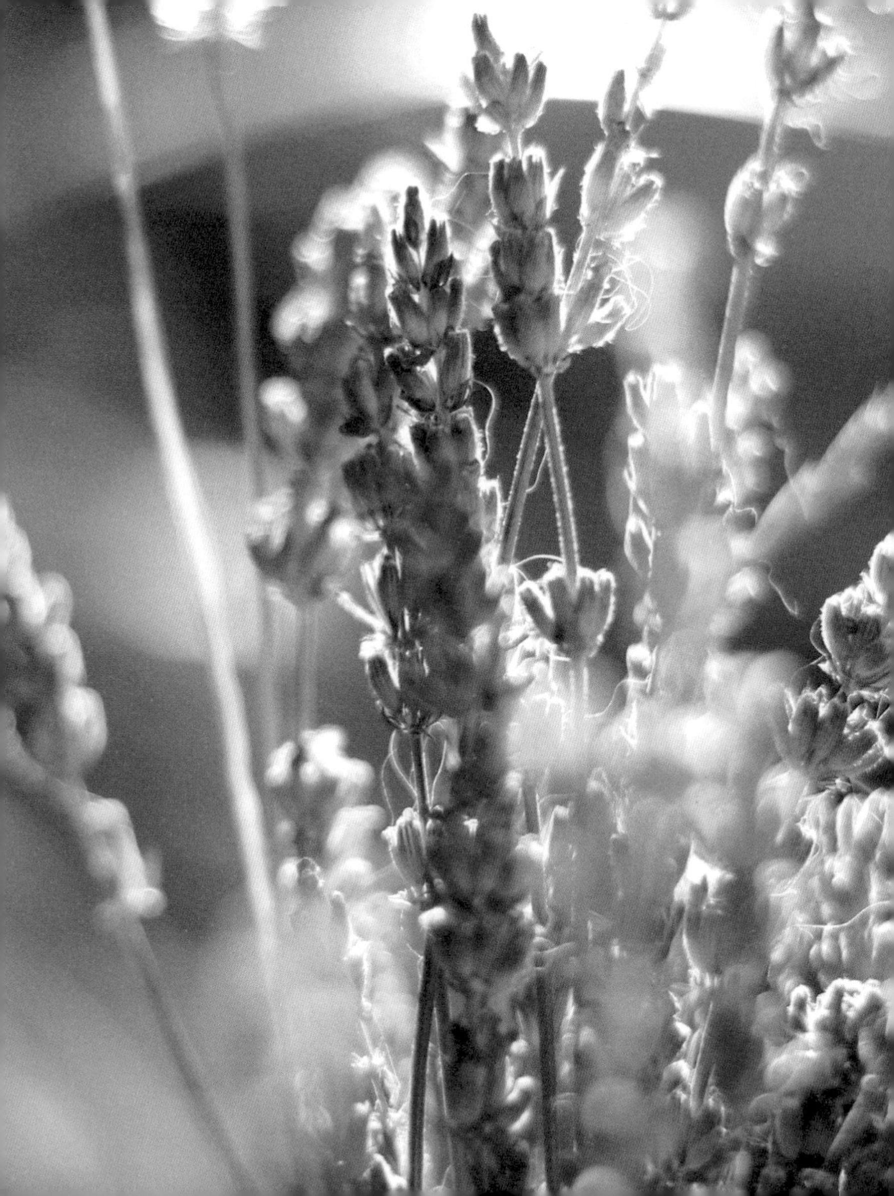

Sleep Recipes

ZZZZZ'S BATH SOAK

A bath is one of the greatest tools we have in the mission to care for ourselves. A bath as part of your bedtime routine is a magnificent addition to a holistic and aromatic wellness plan. In this recipe, chickpea flour will soothe your body, so you emerge from your bath with silky soft skin. With its cocoa butter, lavender flowers, CBD oil and astonishing essential oils, this recipe has all the ingredients for a peaceful and luxurious soak.

Ingredients

2 grams dried lavender flowers
60 gram chickpea powder
20 gram cocoa butter
17ml CBD oil
10 drops lavender essential oil
10 drops petitgrain essential oil
6 drops ylang ylang essential oil

Method

1. In your glass or stainless steel bowl combine the chickpea powder and lavender flowers.

2. Grate the cocoa butter into the bowl. I recommend you chill the cocoa before use, as it will be easier to grate.

3. Stir in the CBD oil, and the three essential oils.

4. Transfer to the glass jar and seal with the lid.

Directions for use

While you are running your bath, add three scoops of the bath soak. Swirl it around with your hand to ensure even distribution.

Equipment & Storage

Digital kitchen scale
Glass or stainless steel bowl
Standard kitchen grater
Stirrer
100ml glass jar with lid

Alchemy Note

The longer you leave this blend sealed in the jar, the more aromatically infused the mixture will become.

SWEET DREAMS ROLLER BLEND

CBD is rightly famous as a sweet sleep aid, mostly since it has the ability to reduce feelings of stress and anxiety, therefore helping us to unwind. It is near impossible to relax and get a restful night's sleep when anxiety is circling us, so marrying CBD and some of our favourite sleep-inducing essential oils is a great start to getting you a better night's sleep. In this recipe, lavender and marjoram invite a sense of calm security while Roman chamomile serves to take you to the next level of restfulness.

If you are fortunate enough to grow lavender in your garden, you can use fresh lavender instead of the dried lavender flowers suggested in the ingredients list.

Ingredients

9ml CBD oil
3 drops marjoram essential oil
3 drops lavender essential oil
2 drops Roman chamomile essential oil

Method

1. Add 9ml of CBD oil to the roller blend bottle.

2. Add to the roller bottle the drops for all three essential oils.

3. Apply the roller ball and then the cap. Shake to blend the vegetable and essential oils.

Directions for use

Apply to your pulses ten minutes before bedtime and take three deep breaths.

Equipment & Storage

10ml roller ball bottle
In a dark glass bottle your roller ball blend will keep fresh for two to six months.

Alchemy Note

Sleep hygiene has become a hugely significant topic in our wellness routine. In a world where we face many external challenges day to day, one of the greatest ways to thrive in this life is by ensuring we get enough good quality sleep. The great news is we get the opportunity to rest every night, so ensuring our sleep hygiene is as good as it can possibly be is a brilliant way to guarantee we are sufficiently recharged each morning. Adding the Sweet Dream's Roller Blend to your bedtime routine will be a game changer for your sleep.

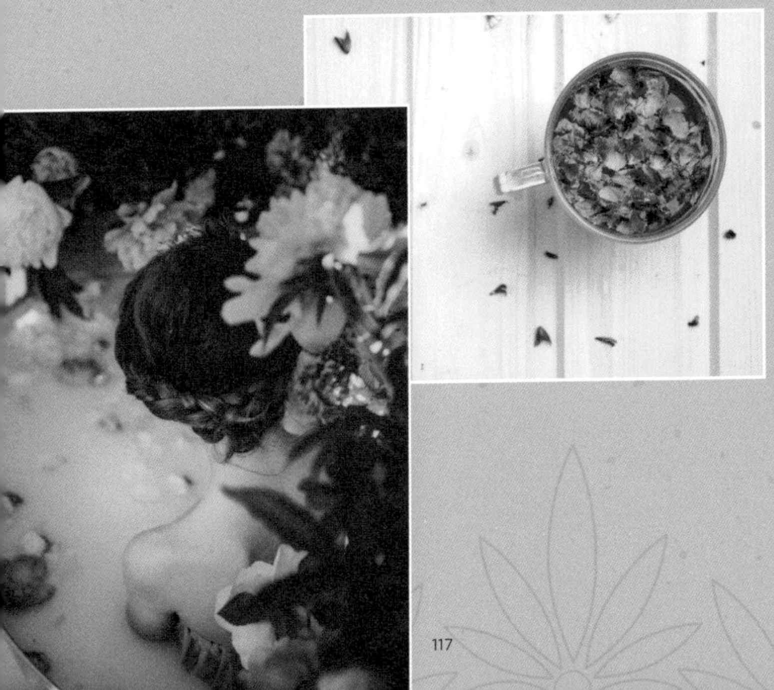

CBD SLEEP PILLOW SPRAY

Infuse your pillow with blissful lavender and relaxing CBD oil to ensure you have a peaceful night. This recipe is also wonderful for children, you simply use it in the same way by spraying a few drops onto their pillow before bed. It only has two drops of lavender essential oil so the smell is very mild and will not irritate their little noses.

Ingredients

30ml lavender hydrosol
15ml CBD oil
5ml vegetable glycerine
2 drops lavender essential oil

Method

1. Combine the lavender hydrosol, CBD oil and vegetable glycerine.

2. Gently stir in the lavender essential oil.

3. Transfer to the glass bottle and seal with the spray application.

Directions for use

Spray directly onto your pillow before sleep.

Equipment & Storage

Glass or stainless steel beaker

Stirrer

50ml glass bottle with a spray application top

Your pillow spray will stay aromatic for up to three weeks if stored away from direct sunlight and heat.

Alchemy Note

Water and oil do not mix so you need the vegetable glycerine in this recipe to help combine these two ingredients together.

Pain Recipes

CBD SOOTHING BODY BAR

A body bar is a great product when treating muscle pain because it's so easy to rub the bar into the areas of pain or tightness. The base of shea and cocoa butters in this recipe allows for a smooth application. These butters nourish your skin while the essential oils and CBD therapeutically tackle the aches and pains we all hold in our bodies

Ingredients

30 grams cocoa butter
10 grams shea butter
5ml CBD oil
5ml arnica oil
Handful of mint leaves
5 drops black pepper oil
5 drops of peppermint essential oil
5 drops eucapluptis globlus essential oil

Method

1. Melt the cocoa butter and shea butter in the double boiler

2. Remove from the heat and gently stir in the CBD and arnica oil, then stir in all three essential oils, followed by the mint leaves.

3. Pour the mixture into the bun cases and place in the fridge to set. Setting will take between one and two hours.

4. Once the mixture has set, peel the body bar from the cases and use as you need.

Directions for use

Massage into the body before going to sleep.

Equipment & Storage

Double boiler
Stainless steel bowl
Stirrer
Four to six smaller bun cases

As there is no water content in this recipe, the bars will stay fresh for up to six months

Alchemy Note

Keep one bar in your gym bag for sore muscles and one in your bathroom for everyday aches and pains. The mint leaves add a new level of cooling to the skin so don't skip them in this recipe. Mint tea leaves will work perfectly too!

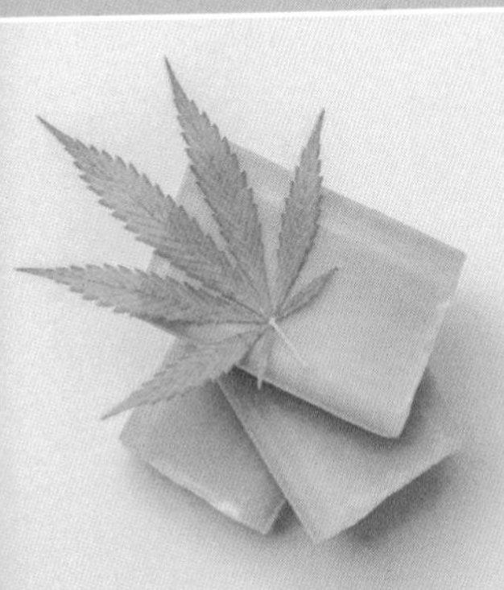

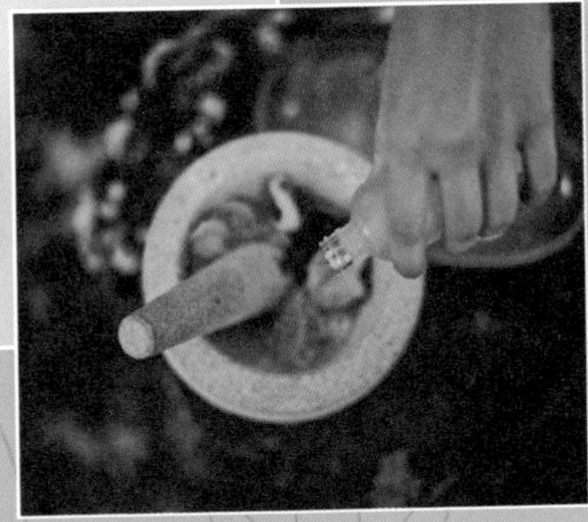

CBD MUSCLE LOVING BALM

CBD oil has generous antioxidant and anti-inflammatory properties, which are the ideal assets for this recipe. This balm is packed with complimentary plant-based inflammatory, analgesic and antioxidant, muscle-loving therapeutic compounds. Together these combine to help our muscles recover and repair after we've worked them a little too hard.

Ingredients

35 grams CBD oil
10 grams shea butter
4.5 grams candelilla wax
10 drops plai essential oil
5 drops blue tansy essential oil
5 drops black pepper essential oil
5 drops German chamomile essential oil

Method

1. Melt the shea butter and candelilla wax in the double boiler.

2. Turn off the heat and let the mixture cool to 40°C before adding in the CBD oil.

3. Remove from the heat and gently stire in all four essential oils.

4. Immediately pour into a jar before the mixture starts to harden.

Directions for use

Massage into the body as often as required.

Equipment & Storage

Double boiler
Stainless steel bowl
Stirrer
50 gram glass jar with lid
As there is no water content in this balm, it will keep for up to six months if stored away from direct sunlight and heat

Alchemy Note

The few drops of German chamomile in this recipe is enough to turn the balm a shade of ocean bluey green. This is beautiful and totally normal. The plant compound within German chamomile which causes this blue colouring is anti-inflammatory, antioxidant and pain relieving also.

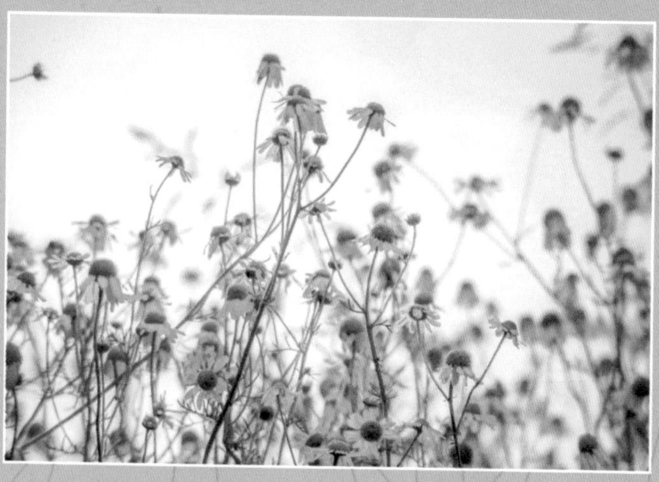

JOINT PAIN MASSAGE OIL

Joint pain is one of those problems we have all experienced at some time or another. Although it can be minor, it can also be the type of pain that slows us from getting on with our day gracefully. One of the best ways to treat joint pain is to massage CBD and essential oils into the area of pain. Not only do the therapeutic compounds in the plants offer relief and repair, but the active message helps to relieve the tension and pain in the affected area.

Ingredients

40ml jojoba oil
30ml CBD oil
20ml arnica oil
14ml comfrey oil
8 drops balsam copaiba essential oil
8 drops juniper berry essential oil
6 drops plai essential oil
3 drops peppermint essential oil

Method

1. Combine all three vegetable oils and the CBD oil.

2. Gently stir in all four essential oils

3. Transfer the mixture to the glass bottle and seal with the lid.

Directions for use

Massage into the body as often as required and especially when you have joint pain.

Equipment & Storage

100ml glass bottle and lid
Glass or stainless-steel beaker
Stirrer
As there is no water content in this massage oil, it will keep for up to six months if stored away from direct sunlight and heat.

Alchemy Note

Joint pain quite often comes with the sensation of heat. The peppermint essential oil in this blend will help to cool that heat efficiently, plus I tend to keep my joint pain massage oil in the fridge as the coolness of the refrigerated blend adds an extra layer of refreshing relief to the area of pain.

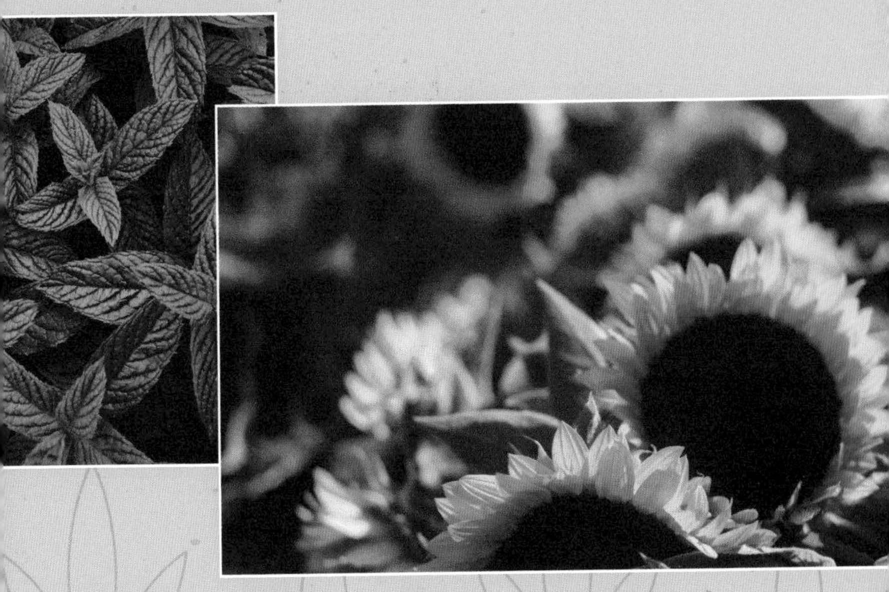

PAIN SOOTHING GEL

CBD oil is known for its analgesic properties, helping ease pain, inflammation and discomfort. Aloe vera not only provides an effective anti-inflammatory action, but its rapid absorption by the skin accelerates the pain-relieving properties of this formidable blend. Combined, these two natural ingredients are a powerhouse against pain.

Ingredients

30 grams aloe vera gel
19 grams CBD oil
10 drops black pepper essential oil
8 drops cornmint essential oil
8 drops lavender essential oil

Method

1. Combine the aloe vera gel and CBD oil.

2. Gently stir in the three essential oils.

3. Transfer to the glass bottle and seal with the lid.

Directions for use

Shake well before use and message into the affected area as often as required.

Equipment & Storage

5ml glass bottle and lid – a pump application is super helpful with this recipe

Glass or stainless-steel beaker

Stirrer

This gel will remain fresh for up to one month, if kept refrigerated.

Alchemy Note

If the area of pain also has fluid retention of oedema, it is worth adding three drops of juniper berry essential oil to this recipe as it is a superb diuretic renowned for being efficient when tackling oedema.

Sex Recipes

SEX CONFIDENCE ROLLER

This sex confidence roller-ball blend is a convenient and heavenly way to support your inner goddess and help to build your sensual sexual confidence. Ylang ylang increases your goddess energy while helping to encourage connection. Bergamot is supportive and infuses a sense of self-acceptance and self-love while the citrusy, yet exotic top notes of Yuzu add a brightness to the aromas of this stunning roller blend.

Ingredients

5ml jojoba oil
4ml CBD oil
4 drops bergamot essential oil
4 drops rose essential oil
4 drops ylang yang essential oil
4 drops yuzu essential oil

Method

1. Add 9ml of jojoba vegetable oil and CBD oil to the roller blend bottle.

2. Add to the roller bottle the drops for all four essential oils.

3. Apply the roller ball and then the cap. Shake to blend the vegetable and essential oils.

Directions for use

Apply to your pulses when you feel the need to tap into your sexual confidence.

Equipment & Storage

10ml roller ball bottle.
In a dark glass bottle your roller ball blend will keep fresh for 2-6 months.

Alchemy Note

I originally curated this roller blend to be used in the bedroom or with a partner; however, over the years I have found that it is a beautiful blend to help strengthen my sense of self-worth and self-confidence so don't be afraid to use this blend outside of the bedroom when you need a little reassurance and self-belief.

CBD APHRODISIAC MASSAGE OIL

Certain essential oils are my go-to for love, passion and a little lust. Rose is the definitive oil for self-love, with a scent to envelope you in adornment, while jasmine brings an exotic and floral aroma that encourages you to feel balanced, relaxed and helps get you into that perfect aphrodisiac mood. I also love grounding patchouli as a boost to your energy levels while also decreasing stress, allowing space for you to unwind. The CBD in this massage blend works to reduce nervousness and shake the voice of internal anxiety.

Ingredients

30ml CBD oil
19ml argan oil
10 drops rose essential oil
8 drops patchouli essential oil
6 drops jasmine essential oil

Method

1. Combine the argan and CBD oil.

2. Gently stir in the drops from all three essential oils.

3. Transfer the mixture to the glass bottle and seal with the lid.

Directions for use

Shake the blend before use. Enjoy your divine aphrodisiac massage oil.

Equipment & Storage

50ml glass bottle and lid
Glass or stainless-steel beaker
Stirrer
As there is no water content in this massage oil, it will keep for up to six months if stored away from direct sunlight and heat.

Alchemy Note

Your aphrodisiac massage oil does not have to be kept for special occasions! I'm a huge fan of using this massage oil as my foreplay ally with a partner, but also a beautiful massage oil to help you relax and unwind tired muscles when self-love is on the menu.

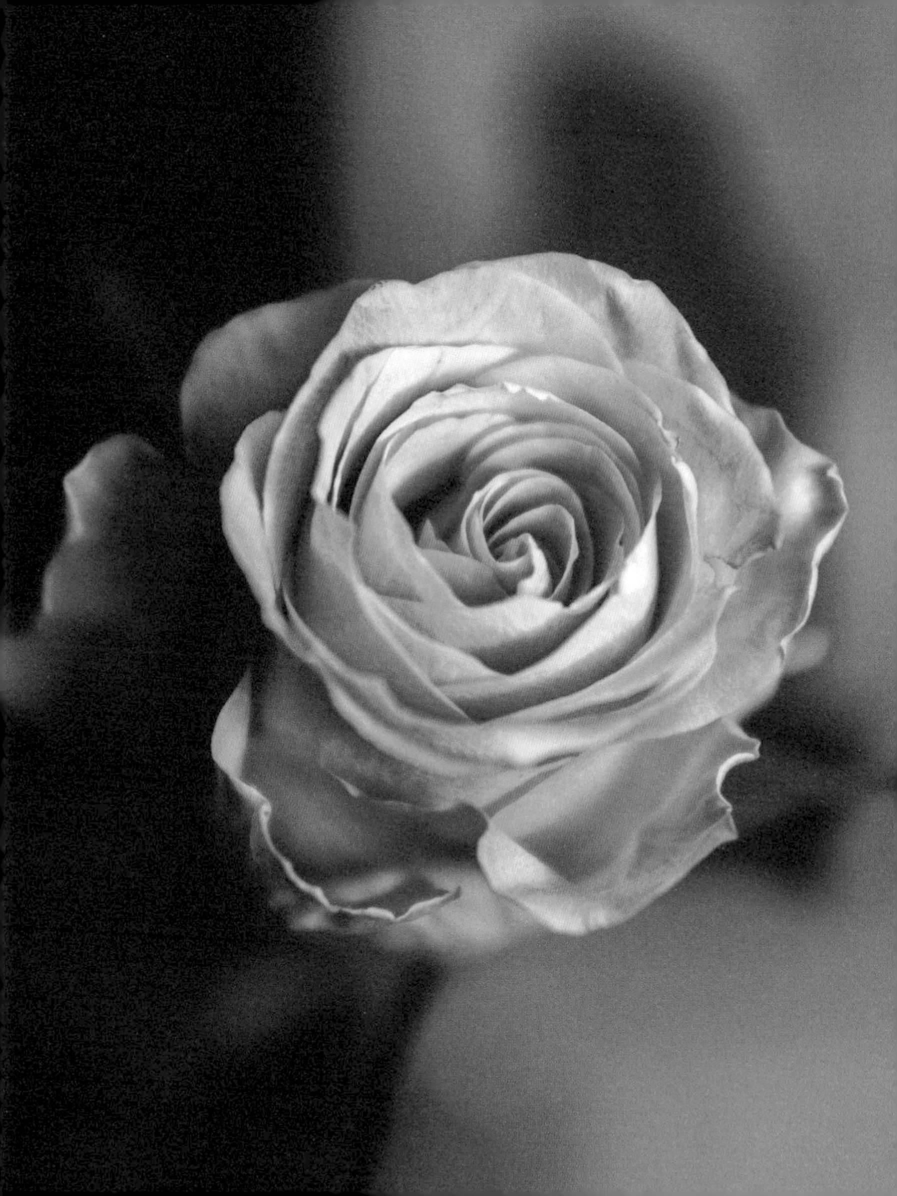

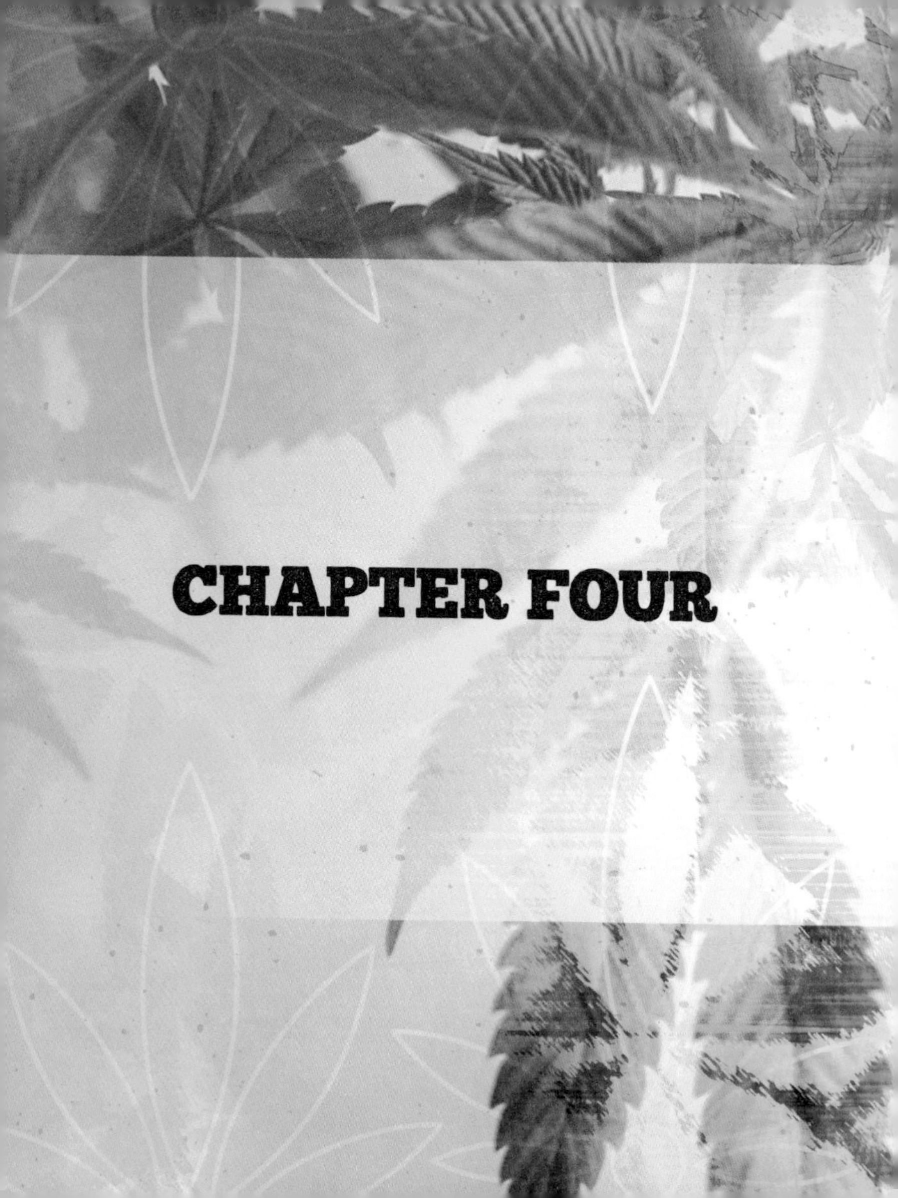

CHAPTER FOUR

The Future of Cannabis, CBD and Complementary Botanical Medicines

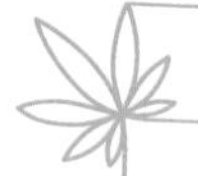

What does the future of cannabis and complementary botanical medicines look like?

First, let's take a minute to understand the unprecedented growth of cannabis and complementary botanical medicines in recent times. Global cannabis sales hit $37.4 billion in 2021 and are predicted to rise to $102 billion by 2026. The global cannabis industry is heading into a progressive period, marked by widespread legalization, innovation and extensive growth. This growth has the potential to fundamentally change how we use plant medicine today, especially within our healthcare.

The growth within the cannabis market in North America in the last decade has been steady but also exponential — more and more states have legalized cannabis for both medical and recreational use. It was estimated in 2020 that adult recreational use of cannabis was worth $12.5 billion and medical use was valued at $5.6 billion. This is expected to grow in 2025 to $30.5

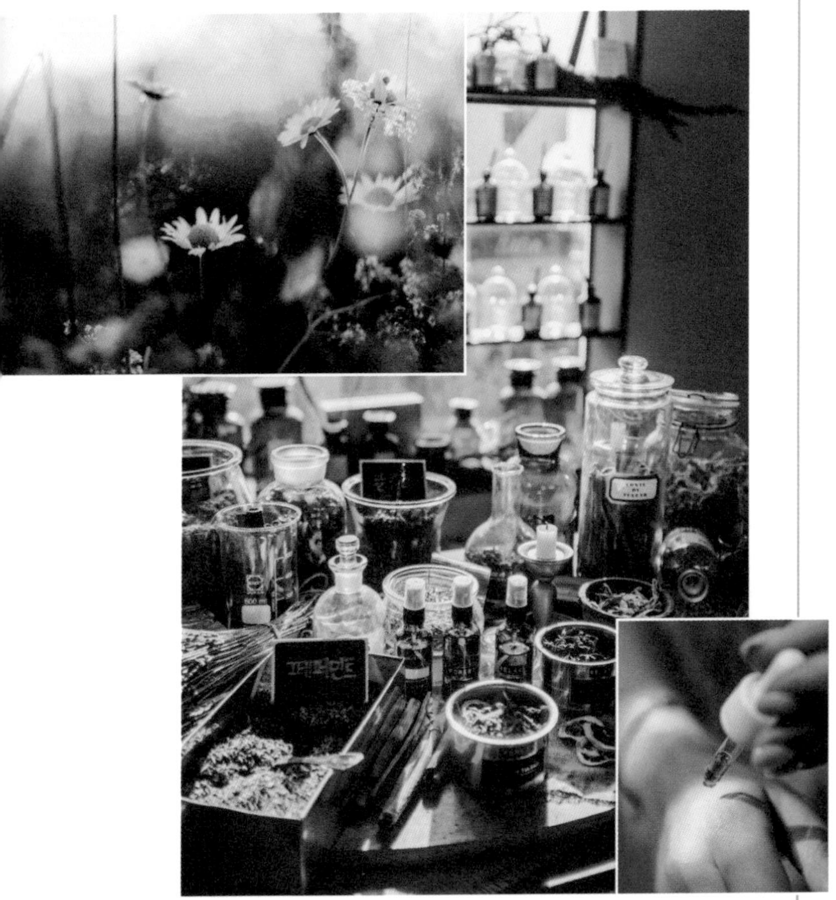

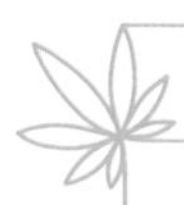

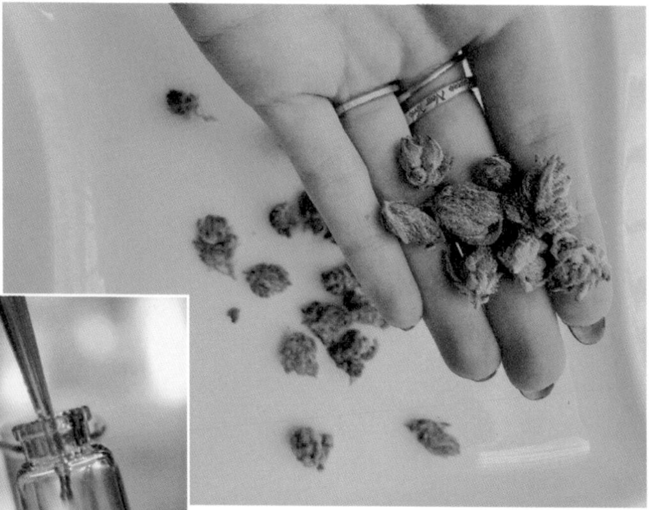

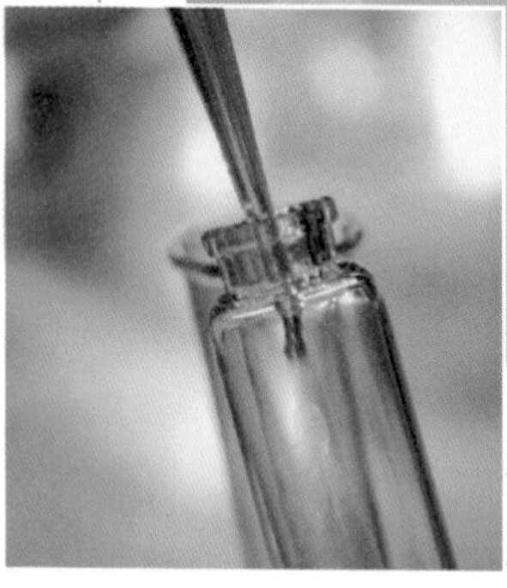

billion for adult recreational use and $8.6 billion for medical use. The European cannabis market is expected to reach $37 billion by 2027 as Germany, the UK and France drive sales. In Europe, cannabis for medical use is becoming widely available especially in countries like Spain, Malta, Netherlands, UK and Austria, to name a few. The legal status of cannabis varies from country to country; some countries, including Spain, Germany and Italy, have even decriminalized the use of cannabis. In October 2018, Canada was the second country in the world to federally legalize

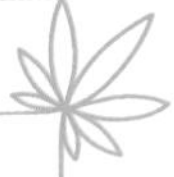

cannabis. In November 2021, retail sales of legal cannabis across Canada reached over 253 million Canadian dollars. Since the federal legalization of cannabis for both medicinal and recreational use in Canada, sales of the plant have increased steadily. Since legalization, cannabis has contributed $43.5 billion to Canada's GDP and $13.3 billion to Ontario's GDP (Gross Domestic Product). This Canadian financial statistic alone is thought to be a convincing incentive for other countries that may be considering their own legal cannabis position.

How do these numbers relate to US citizens? Cannabis is the most commonly used federally illegal drug in the United States; 48.2 million people, or about 18% of Americans, used it at least once in 2019. There are an estimated 3.6 million state-legal medical cannabis patients and there were 3.43 million recreational cannabis users in the United States in 2020; by 2025, this number is set to double. The main medicinal uses of cannabis in the US are reported to be pain, especially chronic pain and nerve-related pain, PTSD, Parkinson's disease, inflammatory conditions, stress and anxiety.

Furthermore, and interestingly, we are starting to see the growth of the cannabis market impact the herbal medicine market. A herb is defined as a plant or plant part that is used in medicine, because of its scent, flavour, or its therapeutic

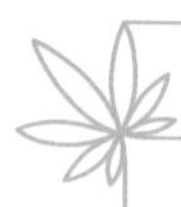

properties. As an example, essential oils fall under this definition. The global herbal medicine market size was estimated to be US$ 83 billion in 2019 and is expected to reach US$ 550 billion by 2030 at a growth rate of 18.9% through 2030. In the last five years, sales of medicinal plants doubled in China, tripled in India and grew by 25% in Europe. The rise in demand for natural medicine across the globe is escalating the growth of medicinal herbs market.

The growth in the cannabis market has affected the popularity of other botanicals not just because of a renewed awareness but because the synergetic relationship between cannabis, its compounds like CBD and other botanicals is becoming utilized and trusted in the beauty and wellness spaces. Although this is true, some botanicals more than others have powerfully therapeutic effects when formulated alongside cannabis. The botanicals which perform better therapeutically alongside cannabis tend to be the botanicals with a similar or complementary chemical profile to the cannabis plant. So, plants that hold their own anti-inflammatory and antioxidant properties are most advantageous alongside cannabis.

So, what does the future of cannabis and complementary botanical medicines look like? The future is personalization medicine. A model which includes plants, pharmaceuticals and

lifestyle considerations, as well as our own unique DNA, is being modelled as our most beneficial approach to healthcare.

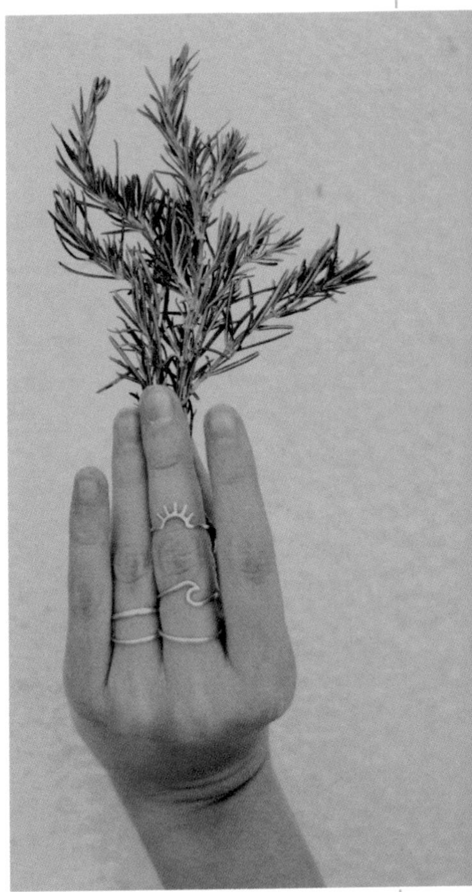

Throughout history — and to a great extent in our modern world — the practice of medicine has largely been reactive. We typically wait until the beginning of diseases and then try to treat or cure ourselves, often leaning into pharmaceuticals. And because we don't fully understand the genetic and environmental factors that cause major diseases such as cancer, Alzheimer's and diabetes, our efforts to treat these diseases are often imprecise,

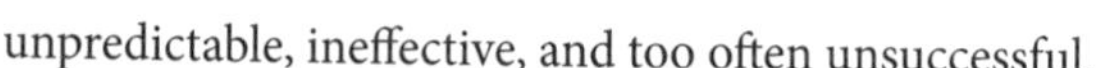

unpredictable, ineffective, and too often unsuccessful.

It can be argued that we currently operate in a 'sickness system' not a health system. Most drugs on the market are tested on broad populations and are prescribed using statistical averages; subsequently, they work for a small number of patients but not for the masses, mostly because we all have vast genetic differences. But how does personalized medicine work? The medical industry is talking about and working towards precision medicine, with cancer treatment leading the way in this innovative field. The aim is to offer a tailored approach to address the unique needs and symptoms of each patient. This concept requires a few vital parts, including emerging technology and our plants. Firstly, genetic profiling (also called genetic sequencing) is needed to help give a clear picture of the profile of an individual patient, artificial intelligence is being employed to define health markers and offer insights into potential future conditions based on the data gained from genetic profiling. Clinical and diagnostic information is gathered and utilized in order to provide a personalized prescriptive healthcare solution. More and more, that solution is including plant-based medicines and compounds like CBD, especially when optimizing the endocannabinoid system.

Personalized medicine is based on each patient's unique genetic makeup. It is beginning to overcome the limitations

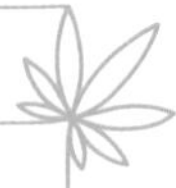

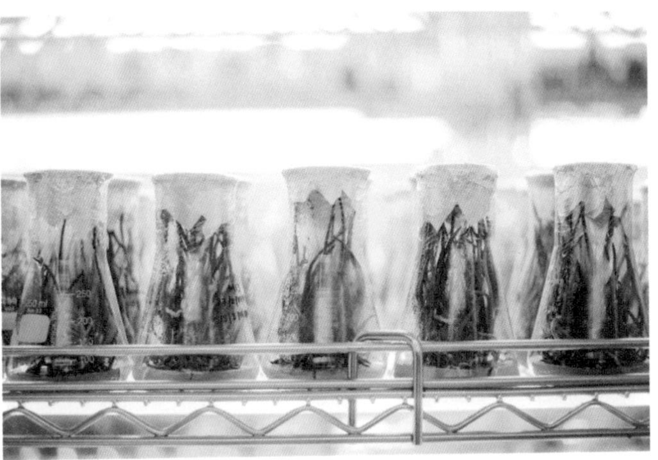

of traditional medicine. This health model offers a shift from the emphasis in medicine being a reaction and now focusing on prevention. It helps predict susceptibility to disease while improving disease detection and pre-empting disease progression. The advanced insights into our unique genetics helps to customize disease-prevention strategies that enable health professionals to be able to prescribe more effective drugs and avoid prescribing drugs with predictable side effects. This will eliminate trial-and-error inefficiencies that inflate healthcare costs and undermine patient care.

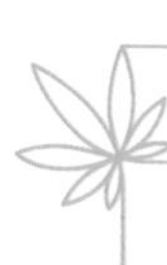

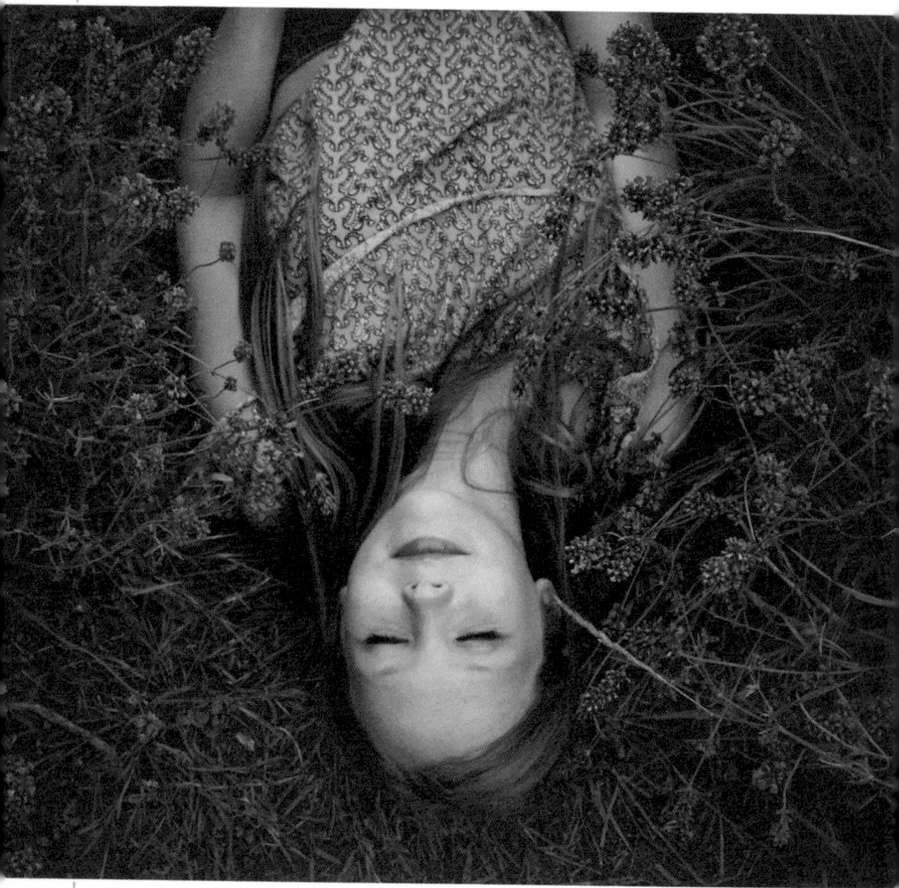

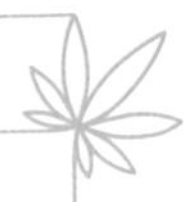

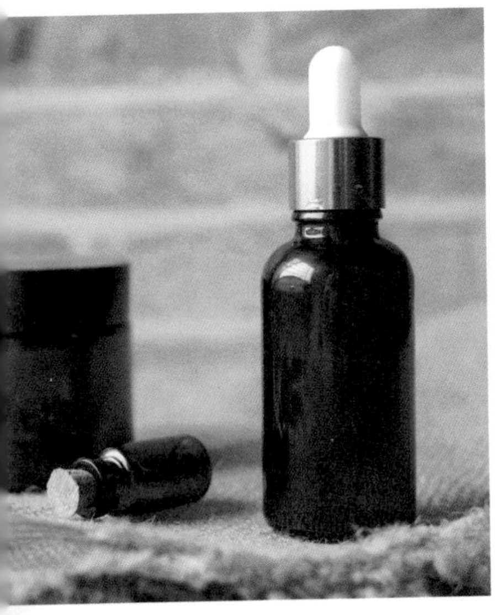

Cancer care is leading the way in personalized medicine. While one cancer drug might work well for one individual, due to differences in genetic make-up, the treatment could be entirely ineffective in another. Israeli- and German-based laboratories are developing a platform and practices that leverage big data and artificial intelligence to better personalize cannabinoid-based therapies for palliative care and cancer treatments. These innovations will allow for the development of therapies that are precise to a patient's makeup and specific cancer.

As the cost of gene sequencing continues to decrease, we have an unprecedented amount of data about our genome that's helping us understand more about our bodies. This area will offer a lot of opportunities for pharmaceutical, botanical — especially cannabis — and tech industries as we move into a new

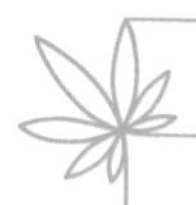

age of healthcare. The question I ponder is, how can we make this new approach to healthcare a reality?

A few key factors need to fall into alignment in order to make this innovative approach to healthcare a part of our day-to-day lives and something we have access to. We need both individual and public engagement as well as involvement from health and complementary professionals. The greatest step will be implementation within existing healthcare systems

Also, the development of sustainable economic models that allow improved therapy, diagnostic and preventive approaches as new healthcare concepts for the benefit of the public. Without this approach to healthcare being developed, with sustainable economic models at the forefront, we run the risk of continuing to withhold affordable effective healthcare from all people.

At this critical stage within personalized medicine, precision herbal medicine is both timely and essential for modern therapeutics, not to mention biomarker innovations that stand the test of real-life practices and implementation in the medical setting and society. Botanicals have been used in a personalized manner for decades, the emergence of CBD and cannabis has simply shed a huge spotlight on this personalized method of caring for and treating our bodies to the whole world. Cannabis, remarkably, has shown us the success of using plants

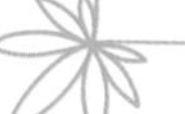

as preventative medicine. The future in this area of healthcare is fascinating and coming at a speed we need.

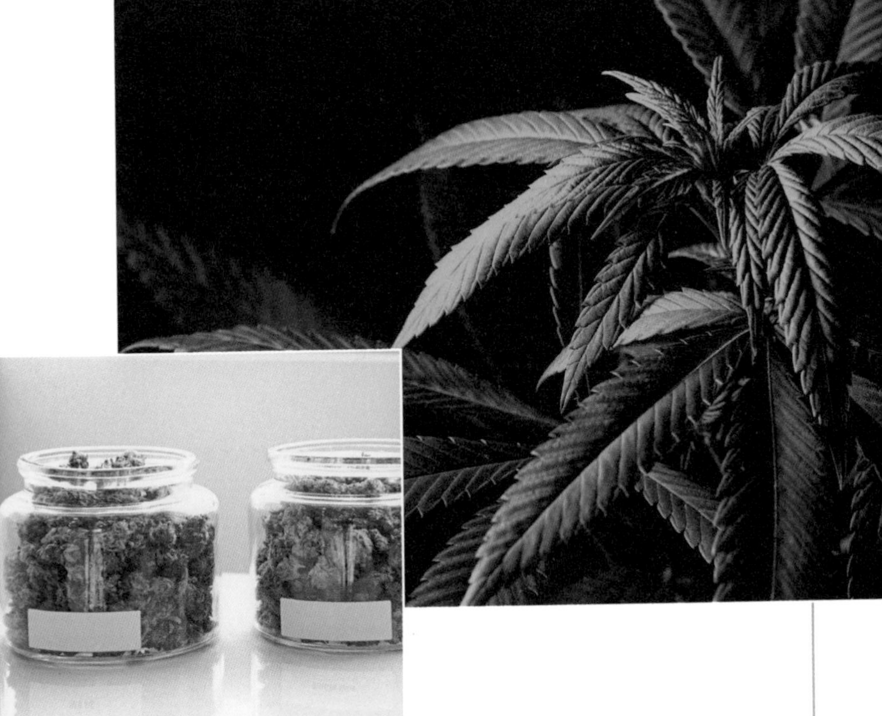

Index

Core Glossary of CBD Terms

Bioavailability
The amount of the substance that enters the bloodstream and can be used by the body.

Biphasic effect
This is a term that describes the effect when a substance acts in two different ways as the concentration increases.

Broad-spectrum
A CBD product that has more than one cannabinoid, but not all that occur naturally within the hemp plant. For example, a product that has had the THC removed is considered broad-spectrum.

Cannabis
The broad term used to cover a group of plants used to produce fibres, medicine, food supplements and, by some, as a recreational drug. This term includes the high THC varieties used for medicine and recreational use. It also includes low THC hemp which is used for CBD supplements and fibres for clothing and other uses.

Cannabidiol (CBD)
Cannabidiol also known as CBD is a non-intoxicating cannabinoid found in varieties of the cannabis plant as CBDa. Cannabidiol available in the UK can only be produced from the hemp plant (Cannabis Sativa L.).

Cannabinoid / Phytocannabinoid
Cannabinoids are chemical components found in the cannabis plant. They include THC (Tetrahydrocannabinol), CBD (Cannabidiol), CBG (Cannabigerol), CBN, CBC (Cannabichromene) and THCV (Tetrahydrocannabivarin). To date there are 113 known phytocannabinoids.

Cannabinol (CBN)
Cannabinol is a cannabinoid found in the cannabis plant. Like THC it is a controlled substance in the UK and should not be found in levels of more than 1mg per container in CBD products. CBN occurs when THC ages. It is mildly psychoactive and is believed to have effects as a neuroprotectant and in reducing intraocular pressure.

CB1 receptors
Cannabinoid receptors, which form part of the endocannabinoid system, found on cell surfaces in the human body, concentrated in the brain, central nervous system and some other organs.

CB2 receptors
Cannabinoid receptors, which form part of the endocannabinoid system, found on cell surfaces in the human body. Mostly in peripheral organs, especially

cells associated with the immune system. CB2 receptors are believed to regulate inflammation.

Edible
Edible refers to products containing CBD that can be eaten. This include CBD gummies, chewing gum, mints and chocolates.

Endocannabinoids
Refers to a protein compound, which is naturally produced in the body. These bind to the same brain receptors (CB1 and CB2) as cannabinoids.

Endocannabinoid System (ECS)
A biological system that all animals and people have that maintains balance or homeostasis. This system regulates sleep, pain, appetite, memory, mood and inflammation. It is very complex and made up of CB1 and CB2 receptors, believed to be the most abundant receptors in the body, which interact with endocannabinoids and cannabinoids.

Extract
An extract is a substance that has been obtained by pressing, distilling, or dissolving in alcohol. For example, hemp is pressed to obtain cannabinoids, flavonoids, and plant nutrients for use in CBD products.

Full-spectrum
Full-spectrum refers to the cannabinoids and terpenes in the oil produced from the cannabis or hemp plant. A full-spectrum oil will contain all of the naturally occurring cannabinoids. This is unlike a broad-spectrum product that will only include a select few.

Hemp
Hemp is a strain of cannabis plant that is grown specifically for industrial uses. Unlike the variety used to grow recreational cannabis it is low in THC and has thick fibrous stems. Uses for industrial hemp include making rope, textiles, paper, bioplastics, insulation, fuel, hemp seed oil and extracting CBD.

Hybrid
Hybrid is a term used to refer to cannabis strains that have been bred to include elements of both Cannabis Sativa and Cannabis Indica plants.

Indica
Indica, aka Cannabis Indica, is a member of the cannabis plant family. Indica plants are usually grown for their high THC levels, but with selective breeding, there are now a number of high CBD low THC varieties that are used by some brands.

Isolate
A pure source of CBD (usually 99%), where during the extraction process, everything naturally found in the plant removed. This includes any trace of THC, terpenes, waxes, oils and chlorophyll. CBD isolate usually comes as a crystal or a powder.

Ketones
Ketones are produced by the liver to convert glucose into energy.

Sublingual
Sublingual literally means "under the tongue". This refers to a method of CBD consumption whereby the liquid is held under the tongue to absorb the active ingredients.

Tetrahydrocannabinol (THC)
The most well know cannabinoid found in the cannabis plant. THC is the cannabinoid that is known for the "high" feeling associated with recreational cannabis use. Many modern cannabis varieties have been bred to have higher levels of THC than any other cannabinoid.

Tetrahydrocannabinolic acid (THCa)
THCa is the precursor and raw form of THC. THCa itself is non-intoxicating but when heated the acid molecule is destroyed creating THC which is known for its high.

Terpenes
Terpenes are aromatic oils that give cannabis (and other plants) their particular aromas and taste. More than 120 cannabis terpenes have been identified. They exist in varying proportions in cannabis strains and are known to have different effects on humans and animals.

Whole plant
A whole plant CBD product is one that has been extracted and used entirely in its raw form without removing any plant lipids, fats, or flavonoids. Whole plant products are often slightly bitter and earthy as they have not been filtered.

Abridged glossary courtesy of For The Ageless. Visit fortheageless.com for a comprehensive glossary.

Additional Learning Resources

BOOKS

The CBD Beauty Book by
Colleen Quinn

The CBD Bible by
Dr Dani Gordon

The CBD Book by Mary Biles

Road to Ananda by
Carl Germano

Cannabis Evolution and Ethnobotany by Robert Clarke

Handbook of Cannabis Therapeutics by Ethan Russo

Cannabis Pharmacy by
Michael Backes

Cannabis and Cannabinoids by Franjo Grotenhermen

The Analytical Chemistry of Cannabis by Brian Thomas

Terpenes by Eberhard Breitmaier

Cannabis in Spiritual Practice by
Will Johnston

Cannabis and Spirituality by
Stephen Gray

For the Health of the World by
Eden Labs LLC

Breaking the Grass Ceiling by
Ashley Picillo

PODCASTS

LabAroma Podcast with
Colleen Quinn

CannaInsider Podcast with
Matthew Kind

Aromatic Chat with
Melissa Holman

Professionally Cannabis Podcast

The Cannabis Conversation with
Anuj Desai

COURSES

LabCBD by LabAroma

LabCannamist by LabAroma

Medical Cannabis Certificate by Pacific College

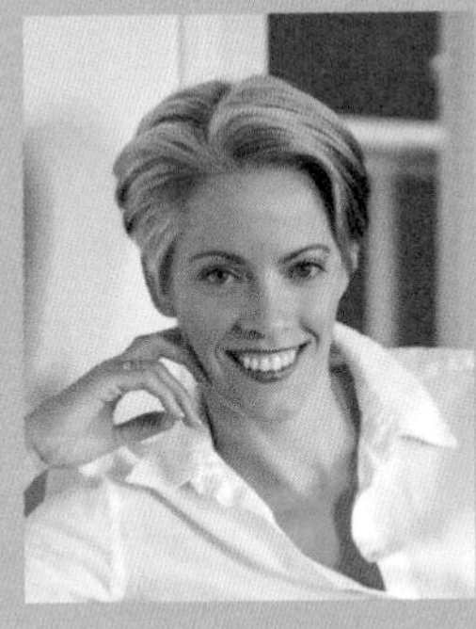

About the Author

Colleen Quinn is an internationally celebrated clinical aromatherapist, cosmetic chemist, author and cannabis researcher. She is driven by an almost missionary zeal to share with you her passionate belief in — and love for — the plants she describes as nature's bounty; the astonishing, complex and beneficial botanicals which have been used since ancient times for their therapeutic properties. This book is her next step in bringing the most powerful of nature's ingredients into your lives for the betterment of your mental, physically and emotional health.

Our modern lifestyle requires our bodies to have superhero powers. Let's feed our formidable, precious bodies accordingly with mother nature's most therapeutic gift, CBD. Colleen is on a mission to educate you about your own internal protection and harmonizing capabilities and how CBD can help feed one of the most important systems within your body, your endocannabinoid system.

Colleen can be reached at:
labaroma.com
lab-botanical.com/
colleenquinnconsultancy.com
labcannamist.com
aroma@labaroma.com

Acknowledgements

To Tania for your kindness of heart and literary vision. Thank you for helping me see this was my next step. To the team at Arcturus, thank you for welcoming me into the fold and entrusting me to bring CBD into the beautiful Elements series.

To our LabAroma community, thank you for your encouragement and commitment to me and the plants. Our weekly calls have become crucial to me as you voice your aromatic questions and next learning desires. Watching you absorb the science and grow in therapeutic knowledge in order to better support the health and wellbeing of your family, those you love and work with within your clinical professions and most importantly, your own health and wellbeing is inspiring to me every day.

To the LabAroma team who support, nourish and grow our community with love and devotedness daily.

To Sarah for managing LabAroma wonderfully as I created this book. It is only with your care and diligence that I am afforded the luxury of escaping into a world of book writing. Thank you, Sarah.

To Mummy and Daddy, thank you for your endless support and encouragement. To Donna, Paul, Kerrie, Gavin, Shannon and Brendan, thank you for making your homes my home and your arms my happiest place.